alternative alchemy

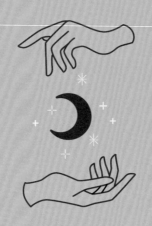

JAMIE HALL

alternative alchemy

Recipes & Mindful Baking
WITH CBD, HERBS, AND ADAPTOGENS

PHOTOGRAPHY BY THE INGALLS

PRESTEL
MUNICH · LONDON · NEW YORK

ACKNOWLEDGMENTS

I would like to thank Willy Blackmore and Jennifer Banash not only for suggesting my treats were worthy of transcribing into actual recipes, but also for introducing me to Sarah Smith, my agent, whom I would also like to thank. I'm very grateful for the talents of Linda Hsiao, of Knotwork LA, who allowed me to use many of her ceramics for photoshoots despite being in the throes of new motherhood (any woman who can make holding a box of ceramics while wearing an infant look easy is worthy of celebration). Enormous thanks to Gemma Ingalls, who not only photographed these recipes but also tirelessly assisted me in all things art direction: helping me with food styling while allowing me to use her sensational collection of props, ceramics, cutlery, and textiles, not to mention her beautiful home (a special thanks to Andy Ingalls as well). And of course, thank you to my family: my husband, Moses, who took time from his own life to work as my assistant during these shoots and provided feedback on the many test iterations of these recipes; my children—Alice (you get thanked twice!) and Valentin, who love me even though I'm always trying to do too many things at once and often have to be reminded to take a second to give a good hug.

© Prestel Verlag, Munich · London · New York 2020
A member of Verlagsgruppe Random House GmbH
Neumarkter Strasse 28 · 81673 Munich

In respect to links in the book, Verlagsgruppe Random House expressly notes that no illegal content was discernible on the linked sites at the time the links were created. The Publisher has no influence at all over the current and future design, content, or authorship of the linked sites. For this reason Verlagsgruppe Random House expressly disassociates itself from all content on linked sites that has been altered since the link was created and assumes no liability for such content.

Text © 2020 Jamie Hall
Photography © The Ingalls

Prestel Publishing Ltd.
16-18 Berners Street
London W1T 3LN

Prestel Publishing
900 Broadway, Suite 603
New York, NY 10003

Editorial direction: Holly La Due
Design and layout: Amy Sly
Production: Anjali Pala
Editorial assistance: Olivia Mann
Copyediting: Kerry Acker
Proofreading: Monica Parcell

Library of Congress Cataloging-in-Publication Data

Names: Hall, Jamie, author.
Title: Alternative alchemy : recipes & mindful baking with CBD, herbs, and adaptogens / Jamie Hall.
Description: Munich ; London ; New York : Prestel, 2020. | Includes index.
Identifiers: LCCN 2020006632 | ISBN 9783791386447 (hardcover)
Subjects: LCSH: Cooking (Marijuana) | Vegan cooking. | Gluten-free cooking. | Baking. | LCGFT: Cookbooks.
Classification: LCC TX819.M25 H35 2020 | DDC 641.6/379—dc23
LC record available at https://lccn.loc.gov/2020006632

A CIP catalogue record for this book is available from the British Library.

Verlagsgruppe Random House FSC® N001967
Printed on the FSC®-certified paper

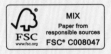

Printed in China

ISBN 978-3-7913-8644-7

www.prestel.com

this book is for alice.

WITHOUT HER IT WOULDN'T EXIST
AND I AM SO GRATEFUL.

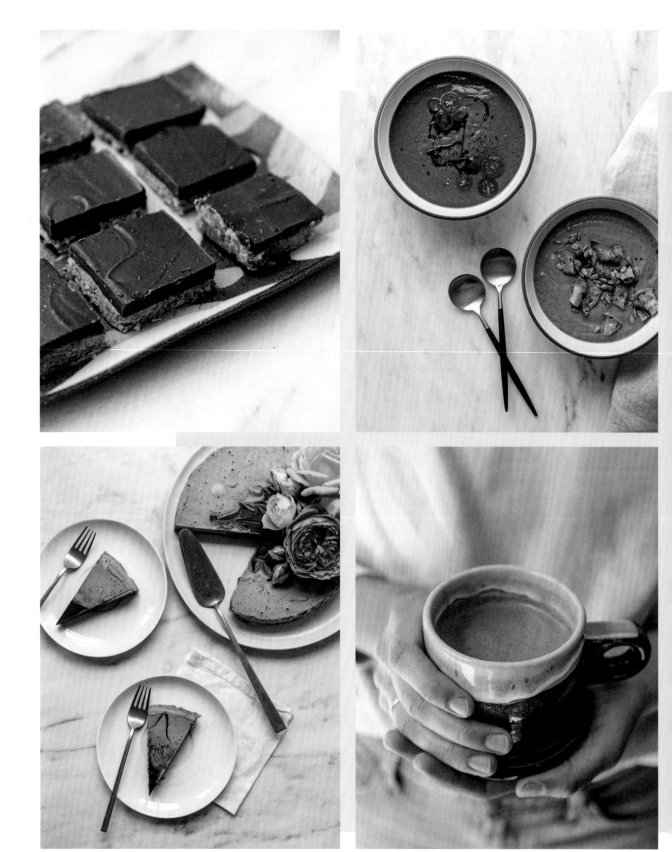

contents

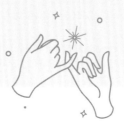

RECIPE SYMBOLS

 GLUTEN-FREE

 VEGAN

introduction

I FOUND CBD AFTER THE BIRTH OF MY DAUGHTER. I WAS A NEW MOTHER, and her arrival was joyful, but also life changing. As time passed, I found myself feeling decidedly *less* joyful. I became acutely aware I was not myself; I had instead developed the sensation I was on mute, or trapped under glass. Long mornings flowed into afternoons, and day and night no longer carried much distinction. I was always awake, it seemed, but never very present. At all times I carried a tiny anxiety in the pit of my stomach—a small but persistent flame I could never quite quell, and when I did get a chance to sleep, I found myself thinking instead of resting, unable to stop the frantic rhythm of my brain. It was distracting at best and terrifying at its worst, and either way, it felt completely wrong. I was supposed to be blissfully engaged in maternal bonding with my baby but instead I was staring at a tiny stranger.

When I got up the courage to bring these concerns to my doctor (terrified she would, at this admission, confirm I was horribly defective and unfit to mother my child), I was instead shocked by her nonchalance. "It's perfectly safe to take certain antidepressants while nursing," she told me without looking up. "Lots of people do."

The trouble was, I've never been one of those people. Not that I haven't tried them—I have, which is how I know. And so I began to look into other things. This was, I should mention, before CBD was so mainstream as to be offered as an add-on for an acai bowl or brewed into healthy teas. In California, when all this was starting, medical marijuana was permitted with a prescription only—and so I got one.

My first attempts weren't terribly successful: I'm not a person who likes to be high (not usually anyway). I tend to have a little fire of anxiety burning at all times which, while occasionally frustrating, also keeps me going, in full type A glory. There was too much THC, I quickly realized, in any of the tinctures I tried in my early trials and forays into herbal anxiety relief.

I read about CBD long before I found it. A brand called Charlotte's Web earned some media attention when they began to provide CBD oil for a little girl with crippling epilepsy. The oil, the articles revealed, changed Charlotte's life, lessening her seizures from moment-to-moment to just occasional and even rare. Clearly, CBD managed to isolate something and tone it down, a refined take on what THC does on a grand scale, and I wanted to try it. As you might have guessed, it worked.

CBD has allowed me to take my mental health back in a way I never thought I would—not because it fixes everything, but instead because it's subtle and lacking the side effects I often fear. It's also easy to obtain: because it doesn't require a prescription I'm not reliant on anyone to get it. The health-care industry is not as easy to navigate as it should be. By finding CBD, a supplement that's available over the counter and at a reasonable price point, I compromise nothing. CBD has been life-changing—not because I drank it in the overpriced lemonade sold by a boutique hotel or because it's quickly snowballed into the next "it" thing, but because it truly offers relief I can control.

I have sold my treats locally for over a year now—mostly to friends and local mothers, but to others, too. I've had a tremendous amount of support from our small community in Los Angeles,

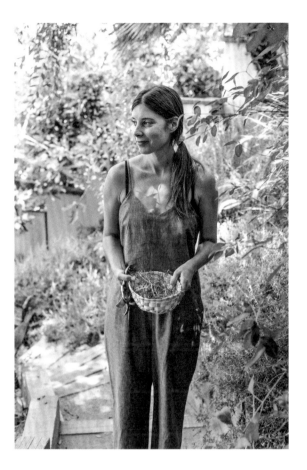

a place with many young families who favor natural remedies. To date, I have participated in a handful of pop-up shops, catered parties, mommy circles, and retreats. I love learning more about it and it's been a wonderful way to meet people and learn more. CBD has allowed me to get a new footing, a type of identity after having children—as not just a baker, writer, or mother but also a very preliminary type of healer and educator on something I've found to offer a tremendous value and sense of community.

What Is CBD and How Does It Work?

CBD oil is a high-cannabinol (CBD) and low-tetrahydrocannabinol (THC) variety of cannabis extract marketed as a dietary supplement. CBD's first successfully documented extraction took place at Harvard in the 1940s. By 1946, scientists had written about its ability to provide therapeutic relief without altering mental abilities, but it wasn't until later that scientists began to investigate how it worked and why. In a (very) simplified nutshell: CBD is thought to exist in several kinds of plants, not just marijuana or hemp, as a natural defense mechanism for the plant itself. When consumed, plants with CBD can change the brain chemistry of the larger animals that eat them. It's likely a bit of a coincidence that it works toward successfully manipulating our brain in a helpful way.

CBD isn't the only plant compound that changes the human brain in a unique way when consumed: Opium, for example, promotes calm and lethargy and was used as a painkiller for centuries in its natural state. Nicotine is part of the tobacco plant and makes for a stimulant. For centuries, Peruvian natives have chewed the leaves of the coca plant, a stimulant, which is also thought to alleviate altitude sickness. These types of plants, in their natural state, are gently medicinal—it's when we start tinkering and refining them that they get a bad name (and often far more potent).

As CBD has gained popularity, more brands have become available. This book includes three of my favorites. The first, of course, is Charlotte's Web. I trust the brand and value its approach tremendously. Originally used as an anti-seizure medication for a small child, Charlotte's Web has a no-frills product design that's often less visually appealing than some of the bright, beautiful new brands I see populating the shelves, but it's a mild-flavored, lightweight oil that has maintained its quality for longer than almost any other. While it is not fully organic, the plants used are and the company's entire farming process is pointed in that direction.

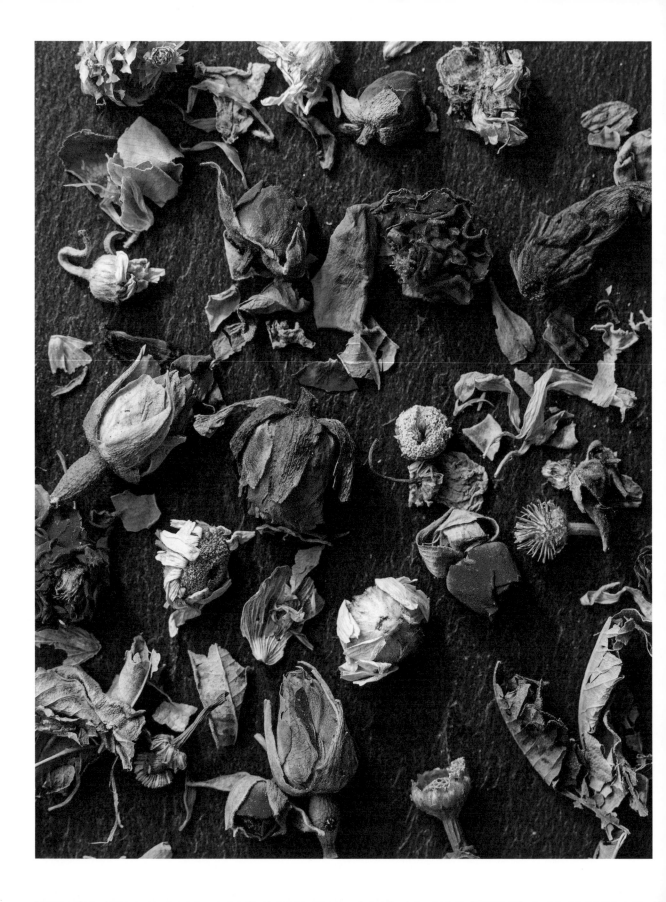

Three additional, newer options I love are Best Buds for Life, which is grown organically and rigorously tested and based in MCT oil; Rosebud, which is also organically grown and lab-tested without artificial ingredients of any kind; and Feals, another tried-and-true brand I trust. All are full-spectrum CBD, which means nothing is omitted and the oil still contains a small amount of THC, though it falls under the legal limit to be called CBD oil (.03 percent).

CBD is not the same thing as traditional marijuana, though its relative newness on the scene makes for a lack of education on the compound. People often mistake CBD for THC or simply consider them to be the same thing. CBD lacks the psychedelic capabilities of THC and the two compounds affect the body very differently. CBD, taken daily, works more like a supplement, with subtle effects that develop gradually (rather than a quick, stoned high).

CBD works with what scientists have now identified as the endocannabinoid system, a network of receptors and transmitters that regulate the body as situations, stressors, and other stimulations occur. If we're hurt, strained, or stressed, our endocannabinoid system produces more or less of what we need to feel better, and it affects everything from memory to activity and appetite.

Some scientists have suggested that, long before we began farming with pesticides and curbing our livestock and animals' ability to find their own food sources, we probably consumed a lot more CBD via the natural food chain than we do presently—which promotes the idea of taking a bit more every day to make up for our depleted, modern-day levels of something we may have once had much more of.

While many people suggest they feel an instant calming effect while taking CBD, the larger results can be more easily summed up as an absence of what you'd otherwise start to feel: anxiety, inflammation, chronic pain, and tension in the body. Because of this, it can work much like an antidepressant, building up in the body over time to offer relief from depression and anxiety. It also appears to work over many doses to dull pain. Topical application offers inflammation relief for bug bites and rashes as well as countless other things, and I'm comfortable using it on my children, too. Brands like Mary's Medicinal transdermal patches and Foria's suppositories and sprays offer relief for everything from backaches to menstrual cramps. I also love CBD as moisturizing facial oil and massage oil. Ojai Dirt Candy is an amazing massage blend that uses frankincense, sage, and sandalwood with CBD that my family found on a trip to Ojai a few years ago. I'm also really into Cannuka—a brand that combines CBD with manuka honey—for lip and face moisturizing, as well as Kana LIT face oil. If CBD isn't readily available where you live it's very easy to order online. Fleurmarche.com is my go-to, and there are a myriad of others.

CBD research is still in the works: New applications and studies are released frequently and there is a steady stream of articles and claims, which can be overwhelming. Research, by design, takes time and CBD is a relatively new focus for most of us, so it's difficult to say with certainty what it does across the board for every person. The attributes that seem unwavering are its natural, gentle ability to alter the body without changing our mental abilities and awareness. CBD is not a mind-altering substance but a body-regulating one instead.

As mentioned above, there are multiple types of CBD. I use only full-spectrum, which means there are still small amounts of THC present (but not enough, typically, to be noticeable). I like to use the analogy of an egg white and egg yolk to properly explain. You can certainly eat egg whites only—many people do—and they offer lower calories and still taste pretty good. The yolks, too, offer something—a higher protein count and filling fats. However, an egg is at its very best when left intact, isn't it? Nature put the white and yolk together and maybe there's a lot to be said for that natural, symbiotic relationship. That's how I think of the CBD and THC grown in hemp and marijuana plants. Sometimes we refine things and they're better, but more often than not we tend to overdo it. I encourage you to find what works for you.

How to Eat It and Dosing

As this book indicates, CBD is most effective when consumed with healthy fats or food and the recipes here are for 15 milligrams of CBD per portion. Fifteen milligrams usually works out to be about four to five drops of oil. I encourage you to make sure you have a calibrated pipette (a dropper with the measurements clearly indicated). Several varieties of oil come with a pipette that's labeled with several milligram servings and can work as a guide.

Many brands of CBD suggest a higher dose than 15 milligrams, but microdosing is my preferred method of consumption. It allows you to gauge where you stand and stop if you feel like you should. The idea of a microdose also works well with using CBD as a supplement, taken several times a day. Remember, our goal here isn't to go back to our long-standing ideas on cannabis; the goal is very different. We're not trying to instantly "feel" anything except calm.

CBD doesn't have the ability to bowl you over like THC might. One of the most frequently asked questions I get is, "Can you take too much?" You can take too much of almost anything, can't you? But is CBD likely to leave you unable to drive or make sense? No. It might make you sleepy, but like I said, it's a subtle enhancement, so don't imagine narcolepsy or anything like it. Just start small and add on bit by bit; you'll be fine.

As for my personal CBD consumption, I like to drink a latte with it in the morning, have a snack midday, and something savory with oil for dinner. If I want to ensure a nice, heavy sleep I usually take another bedtime dose, too. Bedtime doses are nice because they can be mixed with other sleep-enhancing herbs like ashwagandha root or soothing blue butterfly pea flower for added benefits. You'll notice many of the recipes include herbs and adaptogens, because while CBD is wonderful, it's not the only naturally occurring herbal remedy the world offers.

These recipes offer CBD in small portions that allow for higher doses, if you want them. You can use nut milks with CBD combined with a cake recipe that provides more, and top that with hot fudge sauce. Likewise, if you find microdoses are more your style, feel free to omit the CBD in all recipes but one and keep it small.

Occasionally I use pans in a size you might not have, but that shouldn't throw you too much. I offer up a dosing based on the size and amount of people the dish can feed, but I'm no math whiz. I estimate 15 milligrams per serving, but more won't hurt you (neither will less). You can also move the dosing up a notch (many people like 30 milligrams; some like far, far more). CBD won't leave you blindly compromised like marijuana has a reputation for doing. It is not the same thing.

It's important to note that certain items like cookies and frostings, sauces, and individually portioned drinks and puddings are always easy to work with because you can dose them after

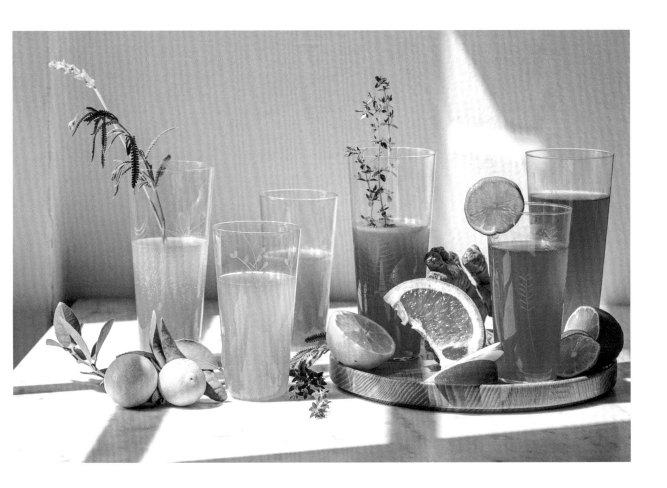

making them. Rather than adding the CBD prior to cooking or baking, you can wait to add the oil once the food is portioned out, offering more or less oil depending on the individual. When it's possible to do this I've noted this in the recipe itself, so keep an eye out.

Herbs, Adaptogens, and How to Cook with Them

Just as pharmaceuticals can offer relief to some, so can herbs and adaptogens (natural herbal substances that help the body adapt to stress and regulate body functions) such as reishi or Chaga mushrooms and Mucuna fruit powder. Find what works for you and hold on to it.

CBD becomes compromised at high temperatures, so you'll notice the cooking times don't exceed 350° Fahrenheit (180° Celsius) and whenever possible the CBD is added at the end of the cooking process. Adaptogens and herbs follow a similar rule and are, when possible, included in recipes that I don't bake or heat up on a stove top at all because they're more potent that way.

Likewise, cooking temperatures vary from oven to oven. Having recently purchased a beautiful, new, very fancy (in comparison to my previous) oven and range, I now know the cheaper version that came with my house tended to cook things much faster. I've also noticed, in testing, this is not a phenomenon specific to me but instead rather typical: The nicer the oven, the longer the cook time tends to be. (I've had great success, when cook temperatures on certain ovens run long, using the convection feature, if available, which circulates the hot air and makes the oven cook faster; just make sure to keep a close eye on things if you use this.) I've tried to be as careful as possible and make notes of this in individual recipes, but remember, for herbs and oils, low and slow is always better than too hot and too fast.

There's also something to be said about food and health. As an underlying principle of this entire book, I'll say simply: What you eat matters. I am a runner and acutely aware that our bodies run on sugar for energy; sugar is not bad, but too much of anything is usually not good. I've never been more aware of that than after having children. Certain sugars and dyes, in particular, make my kids

> "The recipes,
> techniques,
> and ingredients
> are simple . . .
> designed to help
> you feel good."

go crazy; it makes most kids hyper. If we're trying to get our health under control with CBD, it doesn't make a whole lot of sense to fill these recipes with foods that might directly counteract that effort.

The sugars in these recipes, for the most part, are unrefined and that is intentional. While sugar is sugar, these recipes are constructed to avoid a spike in your blood sugar. Sugar can also function as an inflammatory—the *opposite* of CBD. Likewise, gluten is far from bad, and a few of these recipes even have good old white flour (when I really felt like the taste was impossible to replicate or utterly unsatisfying without, because things really should taste good), but for the most part I use an alternative because for many people gluten can trigger other autoimmune issues. This is *not* me saying you have a gluten intolerance and should never eat gluten again. I would never say that. The chocolate I use is always dark chocolate and as unprocessed as I can find, and the peanut butter is natural (and can always be swapped for almond butter or cashew butter, or for those who are nut-free, sunflower seed butter). An oat and coconut flour blend would also work if you're not an almond eater. Above all, these recipes are meant to be delicious and fun. You should want to eat them while also feeling good about what you're eating.

Simplicity and Baking

These recipes are based on a holistic, health-conscious, and dietary restriction–friendly take on traditional recipes while also using CBD as a supplement to promote these same principles. The recipes, techniques, and ingredients are simple, mirroring the lifestyle behind them. Many of the recipes are hearty, protein-rich snacks designed to fuel the brain and body between meals rather than empty, sugar-filled pastries and desserts dressed to impress. My treats are somewhat rustic and always thoughtfully created and prepared, designed to be eaten daily and to help you continue to feel good. They are never fussy and rarely overly indulgent. They're designed for eating while helping the body work optimally.

Most of these treats are made in a single bowl with minimal prep time. Some recipes are vegan while others use eggs, dairy, and traditional flour. Depending on your own dietary needs and wants, you can usually swap back and forth between vegan and non-vegan options without a lot of drama (if you want to use an egg when I suggest flax, banana, or another bonding agent, by all means, go for it—I promise I don't mind). But the guiding ideas never change: Recipes always call for minimally processed, quality ingredients like grass-fed butter and whole milk, free from antibiotics and pesticides. Organic or locally grown options are always emphasized above all others—eat intuitively.

The basics section of this book includes most of the recipes you'll use as building blocks for *other* recipes. I've included a dosing of CBD in these basic recipes, but feel free to omit it if you're using it in a larger recipe (likewise, if you want a higher dosing, this provides an easy way to achieve that). Nut milks create a foundation for all dairy-free baking, and while many of these ingredients can be used interchangeably in many of these recipes, I usually prefer nut-based milks to the real thing. I like the taste, for one thing, but it's also easier on my stomach. You're not me, and I get that, so bake however you feel comfortable.

Making nut and oat milk at home was revolutionary for me. I never run out of milk or panic when it's low because new, fresh, delicious milk is so easy, and (in the case of cashew milk) fast to make. Almonds, unlike cashews, require straining. Cheesecloth works, although for anyone regularly making almond milk I suggest purchasing a mesh nut milk bag (available on Amazon).

Likewise, learning how to make yogurt was equally mind-blowing. I've paid up to twelve dollars for coconut and cashew yogurts, and while some of them are worth it (I'm looking at you, Fermentation Farm), many aren't any better than what I make on my own with the addition of probiotic capsules.

Food affects your body's ability to absorb CBD. When your stomach is full, you're able to absorb more cannabinoids because of bioavailability. CBD is fat-soluble, which means the more CBD that's absorbed by your bloodstream, the more potent the effect. While some research hints at the lower levels of bioavailability offered in edibles (versus tinctures), my own experiences suggest a full stomach and healthy fat make for a more even, level CBD experience.

I designed the lattes to be fast and portable, filled with other healthy herbs to kick-start the body while playing on the idea of this fat absorption—cashews and almonds specifically, with their healthy fats and oils. When there was more of a need I moved into treats: cookies, cakes, pudding, and pastries.

People will tell you baking is all about precision, and some of it is, but that's usually the baking I find tedious and only do when I want to check my reading comprehension levels or impress someone. I like to bake somewhat creatively and part of that is figuring something out—improving it or making it my own (if you try that with laminated dough recipes like croissants or puff pastry you'll end up with an oily mess, I promise).

I began my baking career as an assistant baker, shadowing a very skilled pastry chef while in my mid-twenties, after a series of unfortunate office jobs. The baker I worked with used a single plastic measuring cup for all measurements and practiced a lot of intuition. We mixed flour and nuts to add complexities and when one fruit was out of season we made up new combinations based on what we had and what sounded good together. Nobody ever complained (though I won't lie, I've had some kitchen disasters, but that's part of the process). I did learn how to make croissants, but I've never enjoyed making them as much as I imagined I would and I never feel very good after eating them. As it turns out, I like complex, healthful additions like nut butters and oats because my body seems to know how to process them and they make for a more efficient type of fuel. When my body runs on good foods to begin with, the CBD is only *more* effective—it has less to regulate when my body is already functioning optimally.

These treats run more rustic than fancy and are meant to be hearty and delicious, a healthier take on some standard goodies, and CBD is a healthy complement.

The hallmark of these recipes (beyond the CBD, of course) is simplicity. I always note pan sizes—typically an 8 x 12-inch (20 x 30-cm) or 5 x 7-inch (13 x 18-cm) mini rectangular pan, a standard-size pie pan, or a 9-inch (23-cm) round springform—and for my cookies I use a Farberware 1-inch (2.5-cm) scoop—but here's a helpful tip: Anything will work. Don't have my scoop? Use a tablespoon. Don't have the corresponding pan size? Use what you have—baking times can be modified by watching closely and keeping plenty of toothpicks on hand to check for wobbly centers. I also use a Vitamix blender, but any high-speed blender will work for these recipes.

This brings us to another important tidbit: Ovens and cooking times are finicky things. Cookbooks lead us to believe oven temperatures are far more consistent from oven to oven than they truly are. These recipes were, on average, tested in three ovens and during the course of creating this book I switched from the oven we inherited when we bought our house (nothing special and a total eyesore), which baked everything an average of five to eight minutes faster (and more unevenly) than our current fancy new oven. The other "test" oven was electric, since both of mine are gas. Cooking times generally have a range, but when baking anything for the first time set a low-expectation time and once that dings keep checking every three to five minutes. Almond flour's superpower (beyond lacking gluten and generally being easier on autoimmune issues) is burning far faster than regular flour, plus it's good for the soul to watch a recipe as it cooks. Breathe a little and use your oven lamp to watch the alchemy unfold. This type of baking is meant to be meditative and calming; it doesn't have to define you. And like yoga, it isn't about doing it "right"; it's about doing it the way you need it.

In the event your pan sizes create a different amount of servings per recipe (i.e., a 6-inch round pan would usually yield six 1-inch [2.5-cm] slices), simply do a little math and remeasure your dosing. You can also skip the precise inch measurements and measure out your own serving sizes. That's why the measured pipette comes in handy. Each dose should go from 15 milligrams (what I use) and constitutes a modest dose, to about 30 milligrams—which is more typical for THC edibles that are meant to really make you "feel" differently. (Remember, CBD doesn't really do that in the same way because it's not psychedelic, so I try to think of health benefits over a noticeable change in mental state. You should feel more centered—nothing else.)

Beyond that, I use whole ingredients for these recipes and despite mostly being sweets and treats, these are real food recipes and they will melt, get soft, and start to separate the longer they're left out. Food is meant to break down and it doesn't last forever. A frosting that holds its shape sitting in the sun at an outdoor picnic isn't a frosting you want to eat. I've deliberately made these foods *without* fillers and stabilizers. If you want things to hold up, give them a stint in the fridge to firm them up, and above all, eat them within a few days of cooking them. I've included gluten-free (GF) and vegan (V) symbols on each recipe page to help you navigate your journey through this book.

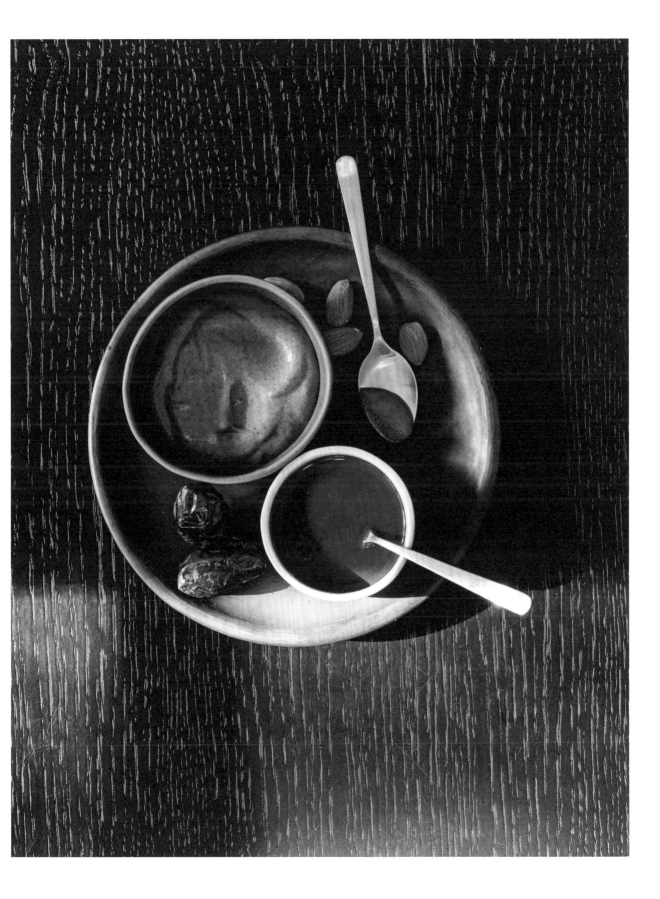

basics

cashew milk

Cashew milk forms the foundation of many of these recipes. I began using it because it's so easy to pull together. Unlike other nondairy milks it requires no straining and, though many recipes will suggest it should be soaked overnight (which is always nice), it's not mandatory for the outcome.

────────── SERVES 4 ──────────

1 cup (150 g) raw cashews

2 dates, pitted

1 teaspoon pure vanilla extract

¼ teaspoon ground cinnamon

60 milligrams CBD oil

In a high-speed blender combine all the ingredients except the CBD oil (we add this at the end) with 4 cups (1 liter) water and blend on high until creamy, 1 to 2 minutes. Distribute into 8-ounce (240 ml) portions and dose each serving with 15 milligrams CBD oil.

Cashew milk will last 3 to 5 days refrigerated and should be shaken prior to drinking.

GF
V

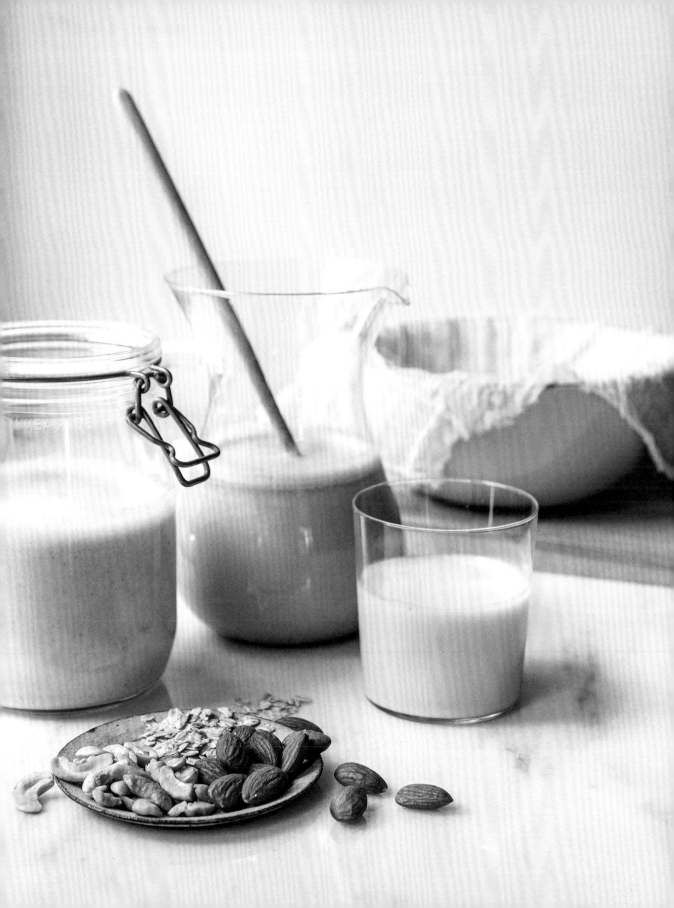

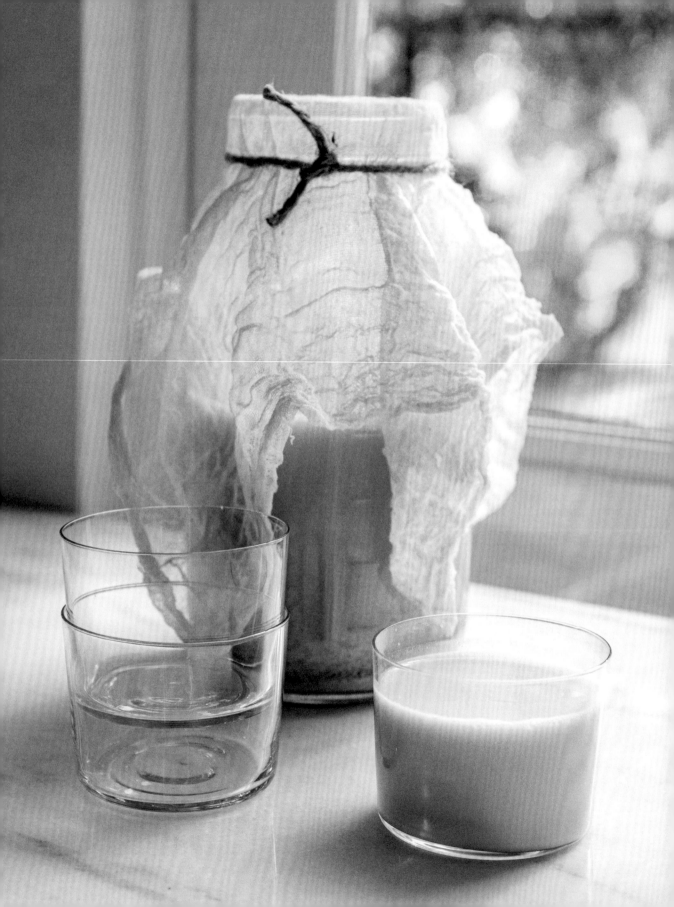

almond milk

While cashew milk provides a creamy, neutral flavor and is simple to make, almond milk has a delicious nuttier flavor. People following an autoimmune diet generally avoid cashews (they're technically a legume, can be difficult to digest, and cause gut issues in some sensitive people) and almond milk is a wonderful alternative.

SERVES 4

- 1 cup (150 g) raw almonds
- 2 dates, pitted
- 1 teaspoon pure vanilla extract
- ¼ teaspoon ground cinnamon
- 60 milligrams CBD oil

Soak the almonds for 4 to 6 hours to make them more digestible and easier to blend, draining the water and retaining the sprouted almonds. In a high-speed blender (preferably a Vitamix or something comparable), combine all the ingredients (except the CBD oil, which is added at the end) with 4 cups (1 liter) water and blend on high until creamy, 1 to 2 minutes. Open your cheesecloth or nut milk bag and spread it over a large mixing bowl, gently pouring small amounts of the mixture from the blender over it, gathering the fabric to hold the pulp with your free hand. (If the cheesecloth or bag isn't finely meshed, it's possible for pulp to pass. A little bit is fine, but try to avoid too much or your milk will be gritty and hard to drink.) Once you've poured the entire mixture through the mesh carefully, give the bag a gentle squeeze to extract all the extra liquid before discarding the nut pulp.

Distribute the almond milk into 8-ounce (240 ml) portions and dose each serving with 15 milligrams CBD oil.

Almond milk will last 3 to 5 days refrigerated and should be shaken prior to drinking.

GF

V

oat milk

Certain things get the limelight at certain times. These days oat milk is far trendier than any other nondairy milk (for good reason: it's more sustainable than many other types). So here's the cool kid.

—————————————— SERVES 4 ——————————————

2 dates, pitted

1 teaspoon pure vanilla extract

¼ teaspoon ground cinnamon

¼ teaspoon sea salt

½ cup (45 g) gluten-free rolled oats

60 milligrams CBD oil

In a high-speed blender, combine the dates, vanilla, cinnamon, and salt along with 3 cups (710 ml) water and blend on high for 2 to 3 minutes. Once everything is mixed, add the oats and blend again for less time, about 1 to 2 minutes, then pour everything through a fine-mesh sieve, discarding the solids and keeping only the liquid.

Distribute the oat milk into 8-ounce (240 ml) portions and dose each serving with 15 milligrams CBD oil.

Oat milk will last 3 to 5 days refrigerated and should be shaken prior to drinking.

GF

V

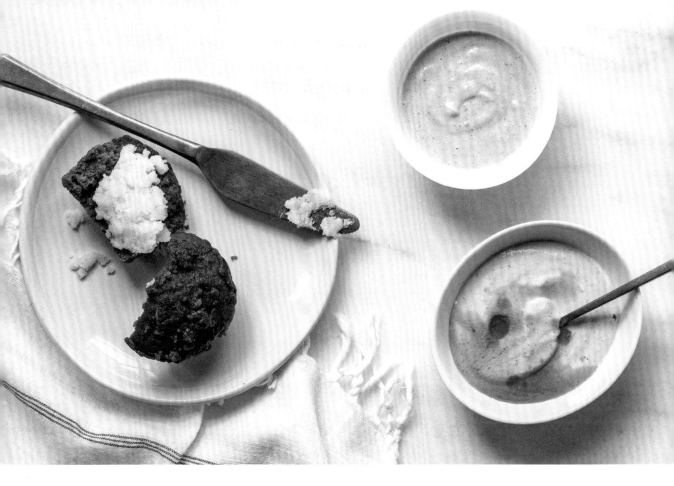

coconut butter

Coconut butter doesn't melt as well as real butter, but its taste is outstanding, and it firms up in a really wonderful way, giving egg-free desserts more structure than usual. It's also easy to make—and anything is better with coconut butter. Really.

——————— **MAKES ABOUT 8 OUNCES (225 G) OF SOLID BUTTER** ———————

4 cups (400 g) dried coconut flakes

2 tablespoons coconut oil

240 milligrams CBD oil

In a high-speed blender or food processor, blend the dried coconut flakes on low until the coconut is processed and turns into a paste, 5 to 8 minutes. Add the coconut oil and blend on medium and high for 3 to 4 minutes. Once the mixture is blended, transfer to a mason jar with a lid and add in the CBD oil. Stir with a spoon. Cover and store at room temperature.

Coconut butter can be kept in a sealed jar at room temperature for about one month.

cashew yogurt

Cashew yogurt makes up the base of several cakes and can also be used as an icing with a few simple additions. It's wonderful with granola for breakfast, too.

_____ SERVES 1 _____

2½ cups (375 g) raw cashews

2 dates, pitted

¼ cup (60 ml) fresh lemon juice

¼ teaspoon sea salt

3 probiotic capsules

15 milligrams CBD oil

In a high-speed blender, combine the cashews, dates, lemon juice, and salt along with 1½ cups (360 ml) water and blend on high for 2 to 3 minutes. Transfer to a glass bowl (avoid metal when using a probiotic) and add the probiotics by pulling apart capsules and pouring in only the powder. Discard the casings. Allow the mixture to sit at room temperature (or slightly warmer—the top of a refrigerator or a slightly elevated cabinet always works well for this) covered with cheesecloth, for up to 12 hours. After 12 hours, taste it. If it's not zesty enough leave it out for a few hours longer, or up to 24 hours; if it's getting too tangy put it in the fridge so it stops fermenting.

Transfer to a clean serving bowl, then dose. If using as a base recipe add the CBD oil with the final recipe accordingly.

Yogurt can be stored in the refrigerator for 3 to 5 days, but once it's reached the desired level of tanginess make sure to keep it cool or it will continue to get zesty.

GF

V

cashew cream

Cashew cream is a pretty amazing thing. It can top nachos or serve as a base for a salad dressing or vegan cheesecake. It's also an ideal place to add CBD—it can hide among the fat for good absorption.

—————————— **SERVES 16 (ABOUT 2 TABLESPOONS EACH)** ——————————

1⅓ cups (180 g) raw cashews

1 tablespoon fresh lemon juice

¼ teaspoon sea salt

240 milligrams CBD oil

In a high-speed blender, combine the cashews, lemon juice, and salt with ½ to ¾ cup (120 to 180 ml) water, depending on desired thickness. Blend on high, scraping down sides with a rubber spatula and adding the CBD oil (unless you're planning to use the cashew cream as a base in another recipe; in that case, follow dosing instructions for the final recipe), until smooth.

Cashew cream can be stored in the refrigerator for 3 to 5 days. If it becomes thicker than you would like, add a bit of warm water and stir.

(GF)

(V)

cultured cashew butter

You can dose this butter and use it as a base in many things and you're set. It can be a medium of CBD delivery for tons of other baked goods. Or you can simply omit the CBD here and add it to your recipes later, because it's amazing as is.

——————— MAKES ABOUT 16 OUNCES (450 G) OF SOLID BUTTER ———————

FOR THE CASHEW MILK:
½ cup (75 g) raw cashews
⅛ teaspoon acidophilus

FOR THE BUTTER:
1¼ cups (295 ml) refined coconut oil
⅓ cup (80 ml) grapeseed or olive oil
2 teaspoons powdered sunflower lecithin
¼ teaspoon sea salt
385 milligrams CBD oil

Make the cultured cashew milk: Boil cashews in water to kill any bacteria, about 2 minutes, and drain. Transfer the cashews to a high-speed blender along with ⅔ cup (160 ml) water and blend on high until smooth. Transfer the mixture to a bowl, add the acidophilus, and cover with a clean towel or cheesecloth; let sit at room temperature for at least 24 hours. After 24 hours tiny bubbles will appear in the cashew mixture, indicating it is cultured. It will also have a tangy flavor.

Make the butter: In a saucepan over medium heat, melt the coconut oil, then transfer to a high-speed blender or food processor along with the cashew milk, grapeseed or olive oil, sunflower lecithin, salt, and CBD oil. Blend on high for 1 to 2 minutes, then transfer the mixture to a butter mold or glass dish lined with parchment (I use a small Le Creuset rectangular dish). Chill in the refrigerator until it's completely firm and can be cut, 6 to 12 hours. I cut the butter into 2 squares to get 8 ounces (225 g) each.

Remember, because it's not made of milk solids and milk fat, cashew butter will melt faster when left out in a warm kitchen. Rest assured it still tastes great, but if you want it to keep the solid buttery texture store it in the refrigerator between uses.

The cultured vegan butter can be stored in the refrigerator for several weeks. Like yogurt and anything with a culture, it will get zestier the warmer it gets, so once you reach a desired taste profile make sure to keep it cool.

GF
V

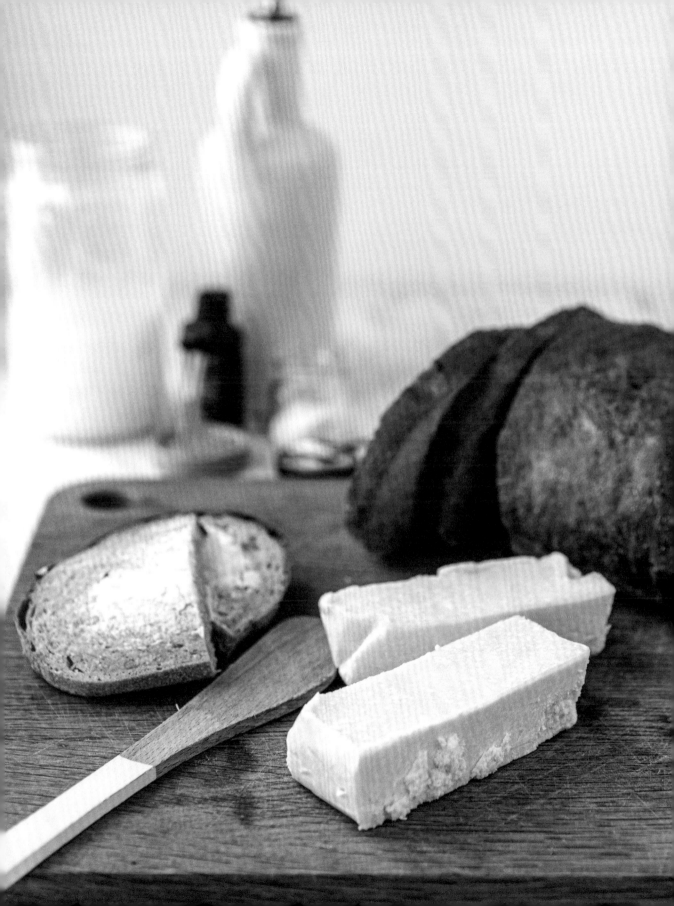

vegan piecrust

Mary Poppins says, "That's a piecrust promise—easily made, easily broken." She's not kidding—piecrust can be fragile. *But*, from fruit pies to quiche, it's so delicious, filling, and wholesome, and I couldn't resist including a butter-free version in this book. Not because butter is bad, but because variety is the spice of life and we should always switch things up.

—————————————————— **MAKES 2 PIECRUSTS** ——————————————————

2 cups (240 g) all-purpose flour

1½ tablespoons granulated, vegan, bone-char-free sugar (it's a thing!)

1 teaspoon sea salt

½ cup (100 g) cold cultured vegan butter (page 28)

1 tablespoon olive oil

270 milligrams CBD oil

In a medium-size bowl, combine the flour, sugar, and salt. Chop the butter into small, cold pearl-size bits and sprinkle throughout the flour mixture, combining loosely into a sandy dough (handle as little as possible with warm hands).

Add 3 tablespoons of ice-cold water, a few teaspoons at a time, gently incorporating to make a damp mixture. Add the olive oil and CBD oil and form the dough into two balls. Wrap each in plastic wrap and chill in the refrigerator for 2 hours or overnight before pressing into a pie pan.

Bake at no higher than 350° F (180° C), watching for browning after 5 to 6 minutes.

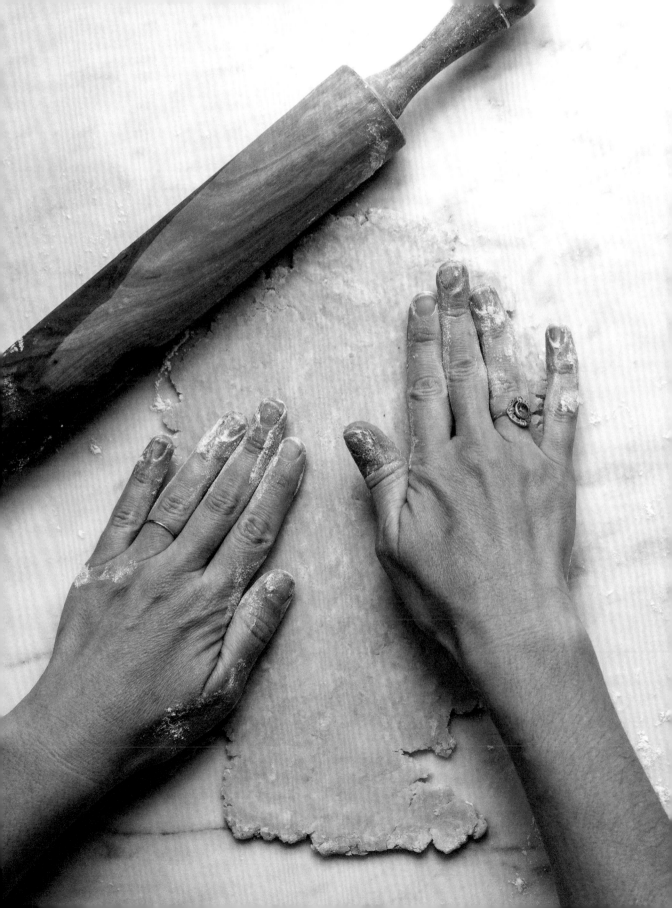

drinks

CHAPTER TWO

LATTES

chocolate latte

My children will do almost anything for chocolate milk. It turns out many of the chocolate milk options they beg for have more sugar than most of the ice cream we buy. I don't mind some sugar, but it's unfair to put so much into a treat that seems less indulgent than a "real" dessert—so we started making this instead. It didn't take long for me to realize that adults like it with CBD, too.

―――――――――― SERVES 2 ――――――――――

4 ounces (95 g) dark vegan
chocolate, chopped

2 cups (480 ml) nut
milk (page 20 or 23)

30 milligrams CBD oil

In a small saucepan over very low heat, melt the dark chocolate gently, stirring continuously. Once melted, add the nut milk slowly, whisking continuously to ensure the chocolate and milk combine. Alternatively, you can blitz the chocolate and milk in a high-speed blender for 1 to 2 minutes until frothy.

Distribute into 8-ounce (240 ml) glasses and dose each serving with 15 milligrams CBD oil.

Chocolate milk will last 3 to 5 days refrigerated and should be shaken prior to drinking.

GF

V

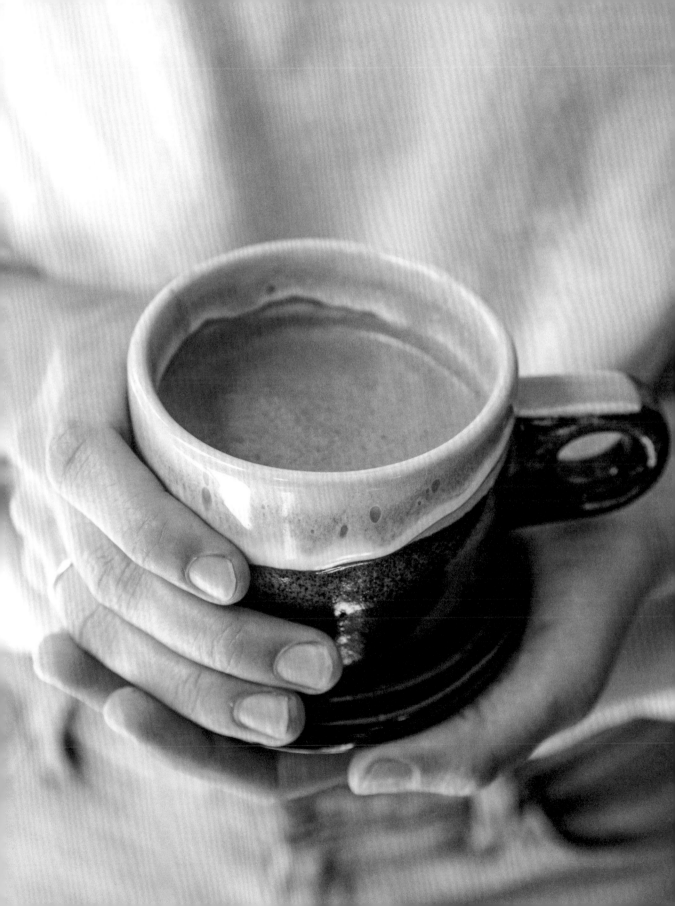

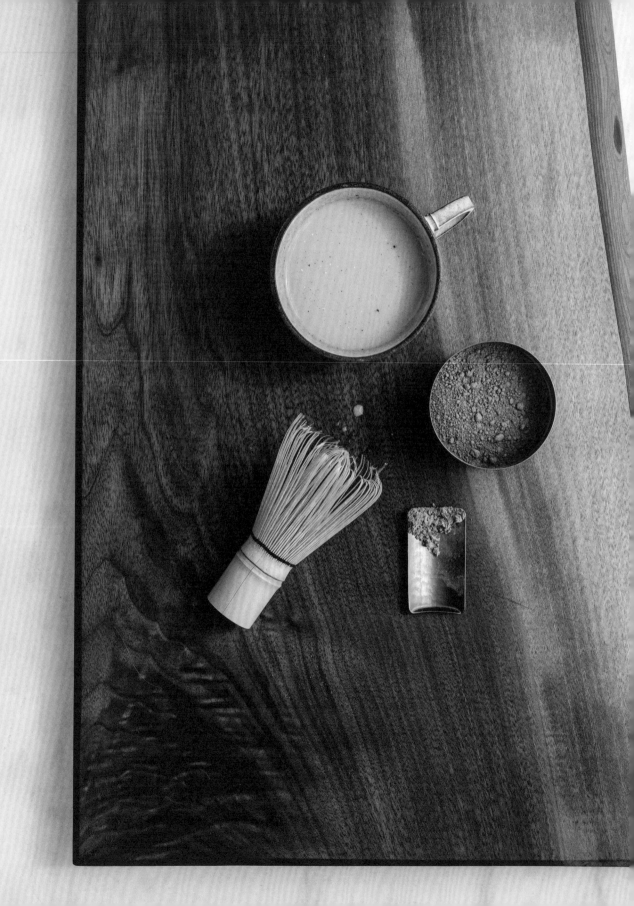

matcha latte

After having my first baby, I found myself unable to drink coffee past noon. It was a shocking blow: I'd once been able to have espresso with dessert with no ill effects, but post-baby hormonal shifts are strange things. Matcha is one of the few exceptions. I can depend on a matcha latte around 2 p.m. to pick me back up. CBD as an additive makes for a nice balancing act of upbeat and calm.

SERVES 2

2 cups (480 ml) nut milk
(page 20 or 23)

2 to 2½ teaspoons ceremonial-grade
matcha powder

4 dates, pitted

1 teaspoon pure vanilla extract

30 milligrams CBD oil

In a saucepan over low heat, warm the nut milk, slowly incorporating the matcha powder while stirring continuously with a whisk or bamboo brush. Once the liquid is warm (but not boiling), remove from the heat and pour into a high-speed blender, adding the dates and vanilla. Carefully blend on high for a minute or two to ensure the dates have blended then allow the steam a chance to escape. Decant into 2 equal portions, adding 15 milligrams of CBD oil to each. Drink immediately.

GF

V

rose milk latte

Rose water is often used in cosmetics due to its anti-inflammatory properties. It combats wrinkles, redness, and acne and just about anything else, but when consumed it's also said to aid digestion issues like bloating and cramping. It has antiseptic, analgesic, and antibacterial properties, plus it's really delicious and soothing. Combined with CBD it's pure magic and is one of my all-time favorites.

——————————————— SERVES 2 ———————————————

2 cups (480 ml) nut milk
(page 20 or 23)

1 tablespoon maple syrup

½ tablespoon rose water*

1 teaspoon pure vanilla extract

¼ teaspoon almond extract

¼ teaspoon sea salt

¼ teaspoon ground cinnamon

30 milligrams CBD oil

In a high-speed blender, combine the nut milk, maple syrup, rose water, vanilla, almond extract, salt, and cinnamon, and blend on high for 1 minute before pouring the mixture into a saucepan. Gently warm the nut milk over low heat, stirring continuously until warm. Do not boil.

Decant liquid evenly into 2 equal portions, dosing each serving with 15 milligrams of CBD oil.

Rose milk lattes are also great cold. You can easily put them into mason jars with lids and store them in the fridge for up to 4 days. Just make sure to give them a good shake before consuming.

You can also use 1½ tablespoons of dried culinary-grade rose petals steeped in the nut milk, gently warmed, for 3 to 5 minutes; strain before adding additional ingredients.

GF

V

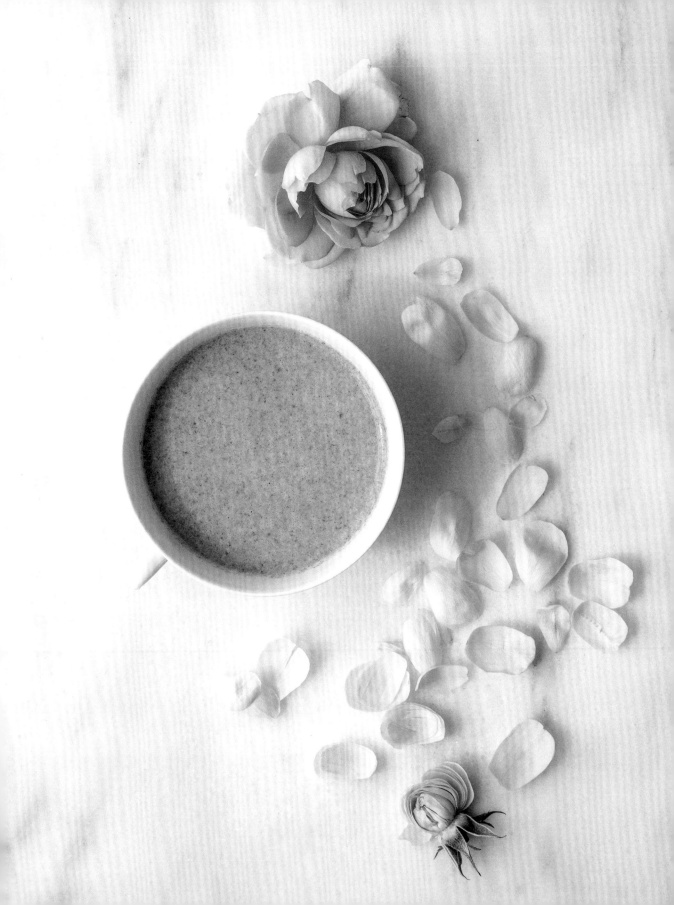

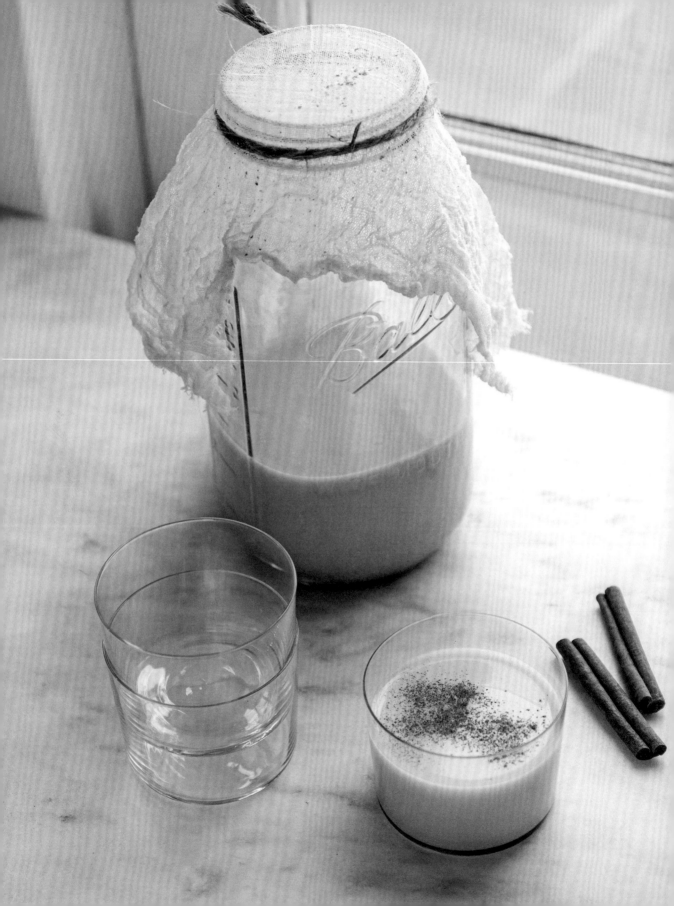

horchata

My husband is Mexican American, and before we met and moved to LA I'd never had horchata. It's now difficult to imagine life without it, which is why I started to make my own. I've never had horchata that I didn't like, but I prefer to know the ingredients. This recipe is just as good as the taco truck variety but made with maple syrup and almonds.

—————————— SERVES 4 ——————————

½ cup (105 g) raw white rice

½ cup (75 g) raw almonds

¼ cup (60 ml) maple syrup

1 teaspoon ground cinnamon

1 teaspoon pure vanilla extract

½ teaspoon almond extract

60 milligrams CBD oil

In a high-speed blender, combine the rice, almonds, maple syrup, cinnamon, vanilla, and almond extract with 4 cups (1 liter) of water and blend on high until mixture is smooth. Transfer to a large mason jar or lidded container and allow to soak for 8 hours or overnight before straining through cheesecloth or a nut milk bag to remove the pulp.

Once the mixture has been strained, decant into 4 equal servings and dose each serving with 15 milligrams of CBD oil. Horchata lasts about 4 days covered in the refrigerator; just make sure to give it a good shake when you're ready to drink.

(GF)

(V)

eggnog

I grew up casing the dairy section for any sign of eggnog. Once Halloween was over I'd start casually checking and by Thanksgiving I had tunnel vision. I could easily drink an entire carton solo—until I saw how many other weird, unpronounceable additives were hanging out with my nutmeg and cinnamon. This version uses CBD for a calming kick, instead of the more traditional addition of booze, but new traditions are good, too.

—————————— SERVES 2 ——————————

1 cup (240 ml) nut milk (page 20 or 23)

1 cup (240 ml) cashew cream* (page 27)

1 banana

½ cup (120 ml) maple syrup

1 teaspoon pure vanilla extract

½ teaspoon ground nutmeg

¼ teaspoon sea salt

30 milligrams CBD oil

In a high-speed blender, combine the nut milk, cashew cream, banana, maple syrup, vanilla extract, ground nutmeg and sea salt (everything but the CBD oil) and blend on high until incorporated, 1 to 2 minutes. Decant into 2 equal portions. Add 15 milligrams CBD oil to each serving and stir well before adding several cubes of ice.

*Almond or oat milk work, too.

GF

V

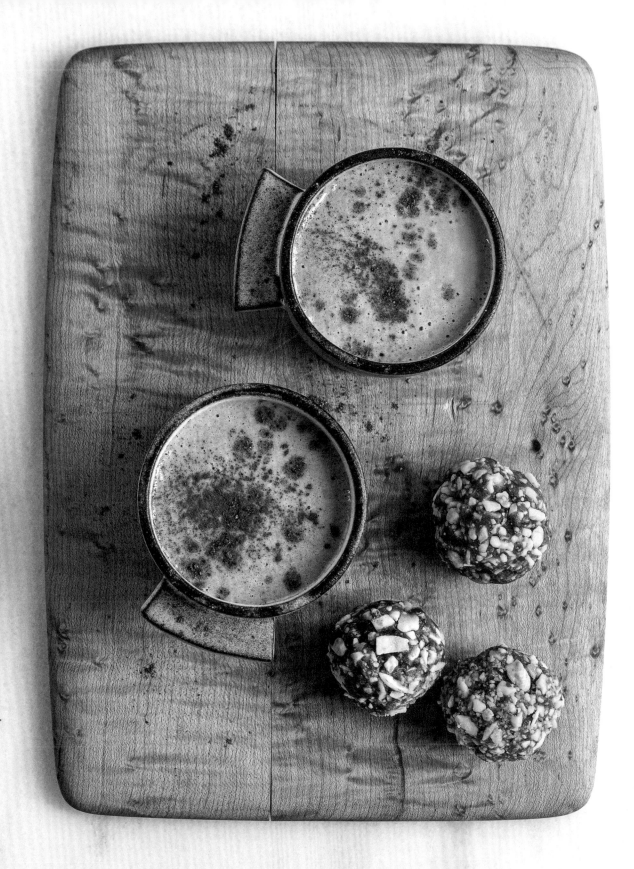

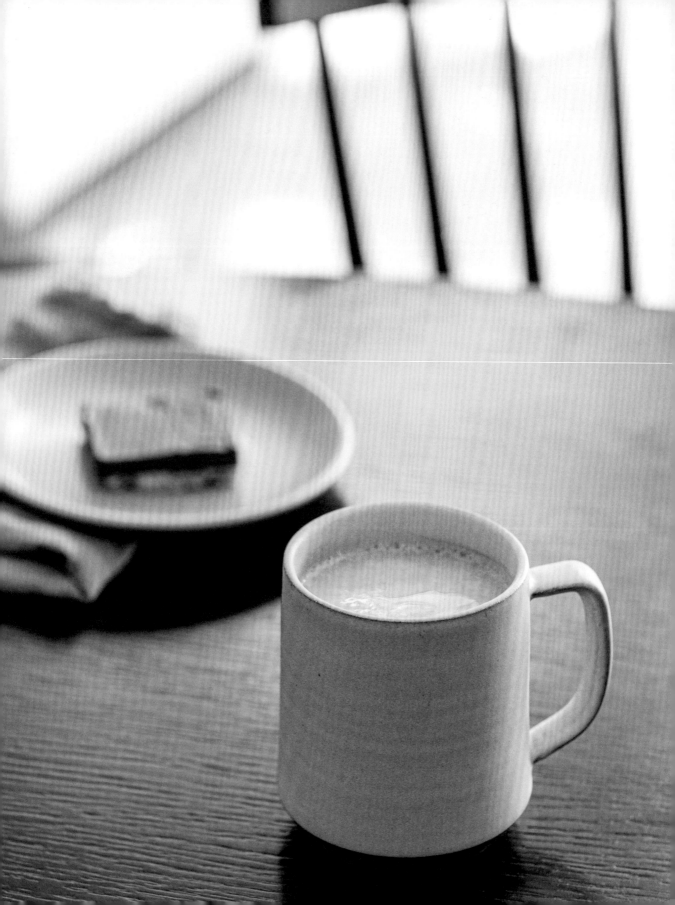

turmeric latte

I make these lattes every day. They're everyone's favorite—a vibrant, beautiful yellow and just delicious. The turmeric is anti-inflammatory and so is the CBD, while the black pepper aids absorption and makes everything a little more potent.

――――――――――― SERVES 2 ―――――――――――

½ cup (75 g) raw cashews

2 dates, pitted

1 teaspoon ground ginger (or a small knob of fresh, peeled, and grated ginger)

1 teaspoon pure vanilla extract

1 teaspoon ground turmeric

½ teaspoon ground cinnamon

¼ teaspoon ground cardamom

Pinch of black pepper

1 tablespoon maple syrup

30 milligrams CBD oil

In a high-speed blender, combine the cashews, dates, ginger, vanilla, turmeric, cinnamon, cardamom, pepper, and maple syrup (everything except the CBD oil) with 2 cups (480 ml) of water and blend on high for 2 minutes. Decant evenly into 2 servings and dose each with 15 milligrams CBD oil.

This mixture is great gently warmed over the stove or poured over ice, and can be stored, covered, in the refrigerator for up to 4 days. Shake before drinking.

GF

V

blue butterfly tea latte

Butterfly pea tea is a beautiful, blue-to-purple tea. In Los Angeles, my local herb shop, Wild Terra, keeps a lovely blend of blue butterfly pea and chai teas on hand, but there are other versions available online (you could also combine the dried blooms, which are fairly common, with a chai tea on your own for a DIY combo). Blue butterfly pea has amazing pH properties. Adding some lemon juice makes it violet; hibiscus flower turns it bright red. Go nuts.

———————————————— SERVES 2 ————————————————

1½ tablespoons blue butterfly pea chai tea

1 cup (240 ml) nut milk (page 20 or 23)

1 tablespoon maple syrup

1 teaspoon pure vanilla extract

30 milligrams CBD oil

Steep the tea in 1 cup (240 ml) hot water for 5 to 10 minutes before draining out the dregs. In a saucepan over medium-low heat, combine the brewed tea with the nut milk and warm gently, adding the maple syrup and vanilla while whisking continuously. Do not boil.

Decant the tea into equal portions and dose each with 15 milligrams CBD oil. Drink immediately.

GF
V

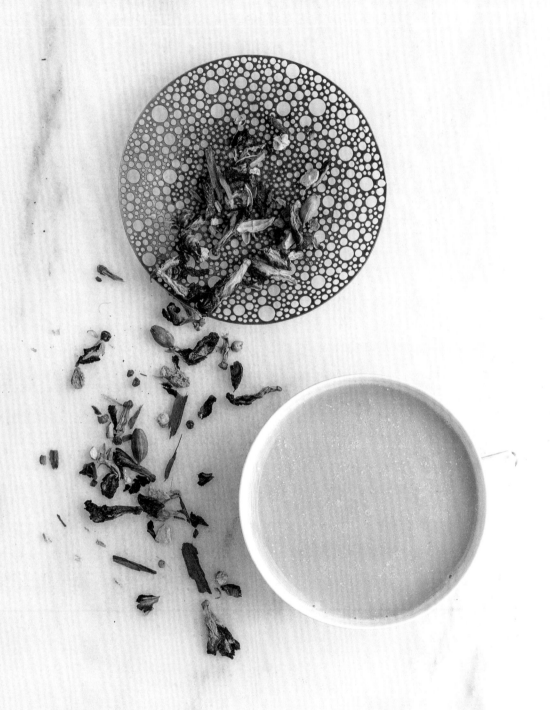

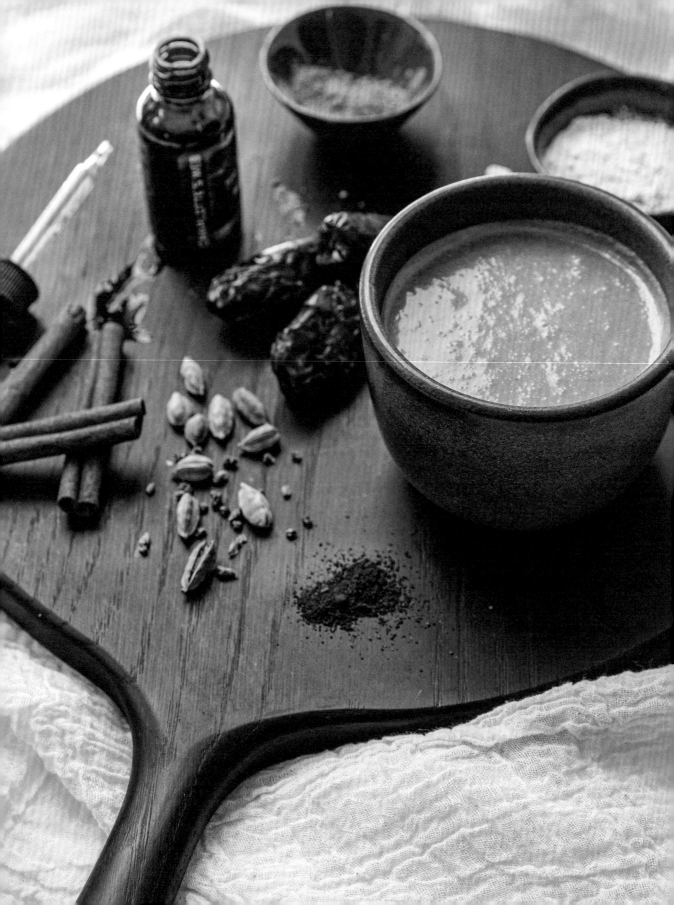

black sheep latte

I said everyone's favorite latte is turmeric, but that's not entirely true. I have one customer who always prefers this cocoa and ashwagandha infusion, but really, they were created to work as night and day drinks—the turmeric in the morning, and ashwagandha, which supports hormone and sleep, for evening. That being said, I love this one with coffee or a shot of espresso, which also makes the CBD easy to absorb, so whatever works. It's always delicious.

—————— SERVES 2 ——————

½ cup (75 g) raw cashews

2 dates, pitted

1 tablespoon cocoa powder

½ teaspoon ashwagandha root powder

¼ teaspoon ground cinnamon

¼ teaspoon ground cardamom

Pinch of cayenne pepper

30 milligrams CBD oil

In a high-speed blender, combine the cashews, dates, cocoa powder, ashwagandha root powder, cinnamon, cardamom and cayenne pepper with 2 cups (480 ml) water and blend on high for 2 to 3 minutes, making sure the dates and cashews are incorporated. Decant into 2 equal servings and dose each with 15 milligrams CBD oil. It's good in the refrigerator for up to 5 days and should be shaken before drinking.

GF

V

✳

turmeric, ginger, and maple tonic

This tonic is our remedy for an upset stomach, but it's so delicious we also started using it as a nonalcoholic cocktail at parties by dressing it up with a garnish or two. Fresh thyme smells amazing and perfectly complements the lemon, while the fresh black pepper gives it a kick and also helps with the body's absorption of not only the CBD but also ginger and turmeric.

SERVES 4

1½ teaspoons ground ginger, or a peeled 2-inch (5-cm) knob of fresh ginger, roughly chopped

2 teaspoons ground turmeric, or a peeled 5-inch (13-cm) piece of fresh turmeric root, roughly chopped

½ cup (120 ml) maple syrup

½ cup (120 ml) fresh lemon juice, from about 2 to 3 lemons

10 ounces (300 ml) carbonated water

60 milligrams CBD oil

Thinly sliced fresh ginger and turmeric, for serving (optional)

In a medium-size pot, boil 3 cups (720 ml) of water. Add the ginger and turmeric and remove from the heat. Stir in the maple syrup and set the mixture aside, allowing it to cool to room temperature. Once cooled, stir in the lemon juice and refrigerate the entire mixture for 3 to 5 hours before straining it through a nut milk bag or fine-mesh sieve, discarding the solids.

To serve, combine with carbonated water and decant into 4 equal servings before adding 15 milligrams CBD oil to each. Garnish with thinly sliced fresh ginger and turmeric, if using.

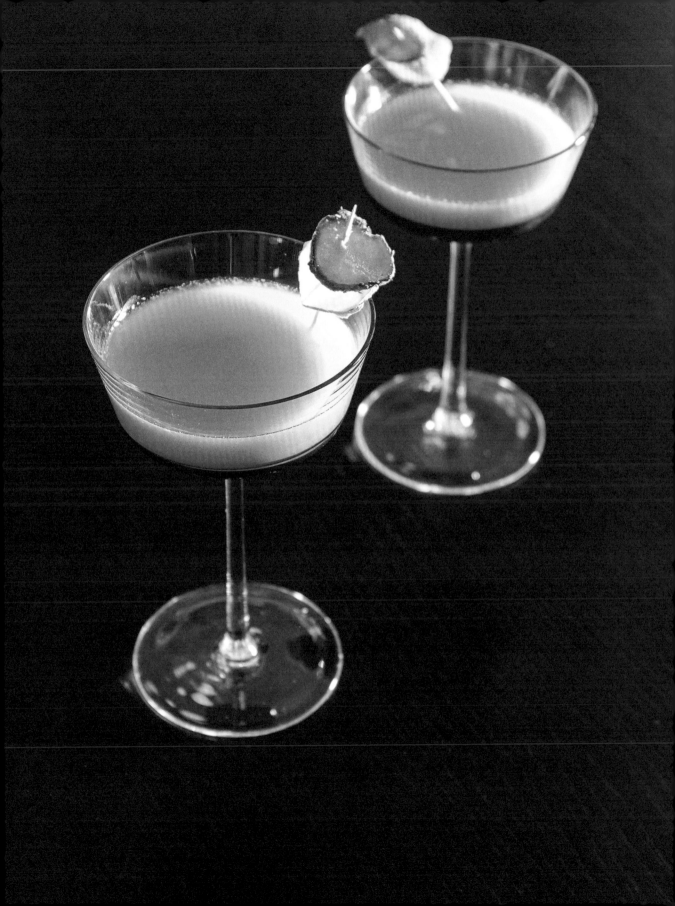

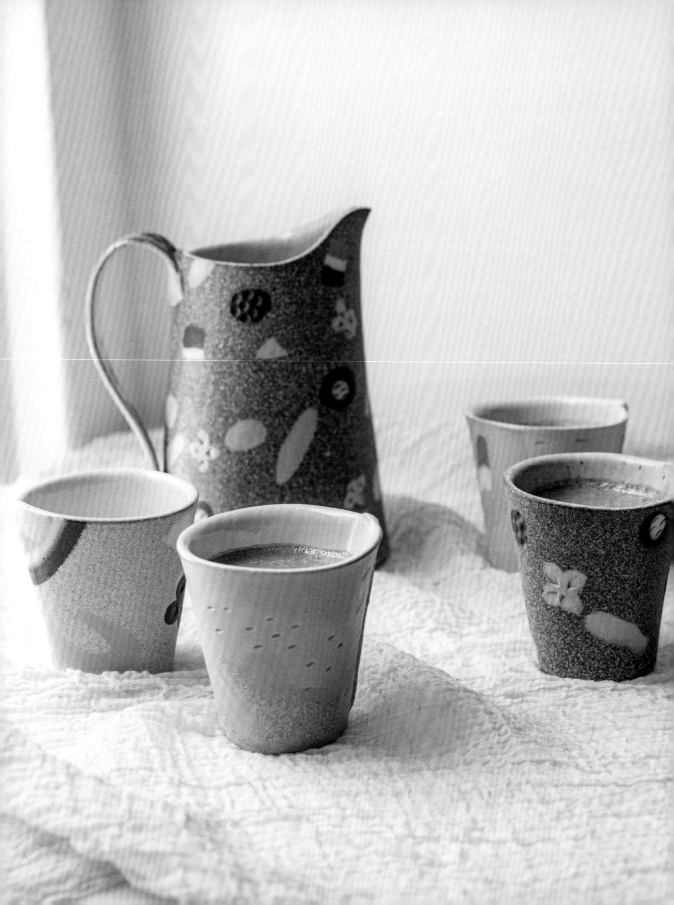

reishi hot chocolate tonic

Adaptogenic mushrooms are not to be confused with the "magic" variety, just like CBD shouldn't be confused with traditional "weed." Adaptogens (which can be mushrooms or a handful of other herbs and pollens) help the body cope with stress and aptly "adapt" to different emotional and physical needs as our environment and mental states change throughout the day, hour, etc. They're a quick way to improve energy, focus, and our immune system.

—————————————— SERVES 2 ——————————————

4 ounces (95 g) dark vegan chocolate, coarsely chopped

2 cups (480 ml) cashew milk, divided (page 20)

2 tablespoons dried reishi mushroom powder

30 milligrams CBD oil

2 tablespoons coconut cream (optional)

Chocolate shavings (optional)

In a small saucepan over low heat, gently heat the dark chocolate, stirring continuously as it melts down. Once it begins to melt, add 1 cup (240 ml) of the cashew milk and whisk until the milk is hot but not boiling, then remove from the heat. The chocolate won't blend completely, but you can now use a rubber spatula or spoon to scrape the chocolate from the bottom of the pan and transfer the mixture to a high-speed blender. Add the remaining cup of cashew milk along with the reishi powder and blend on high for about 1 minute.

Transfer the mixture to 2 large mugs, adding 15 milligrams of CBD oil per drink. You can drink them as is, or garnish the hot chocolate with a dollop of coconut cream and chocolate shavings—you can use bits of any leftover coarsely chopped chocolate, or use a vegetable peeler to scrape off a few curls from a chocolate bar.

GF

V

mucuna chocolate soda

My mother and brother are steadfastly committed to chocolate malts. The last time my mom visited I introduced her not only to CBD but also to an adaptogenic chocolate malted soda using *Mucuna pruriens* (which can be purchased on Amazon or at most health food markets in the supplements section). *Mucuna pruriens*—which, in this recipe, comes from the almond butter ice cream—is a naturally calming adaptogen that helps promote mental clarity and provide energy. This drink tastes as decadent as a true malt but does so much more for you.

SERVES 2

2 servings hot fudge (page 168)

2 scoops chocolate almond butter ice cream (page 165)

30 milligrams CBD oil

10 ounces (300 ml) carbonated water

2 tablespoons maple syrup

1 double shot of espresso (optional)

To prepare the sodas, swirl hot fudge on the sides and at the bottom of 2 pint glasses. Scoop 1 large scoop of ice cream into each large glass. Add 15 milligrams CBD to each glass, along with 5 ounces of the carbonated water and a tablespoon of maple syrup on top of each soda.

I like to eat my chocolate soda with a spoon. If you're a coffee drinker, try a double shot of espresso poured on top. It's amazing. I promise.

GF

V

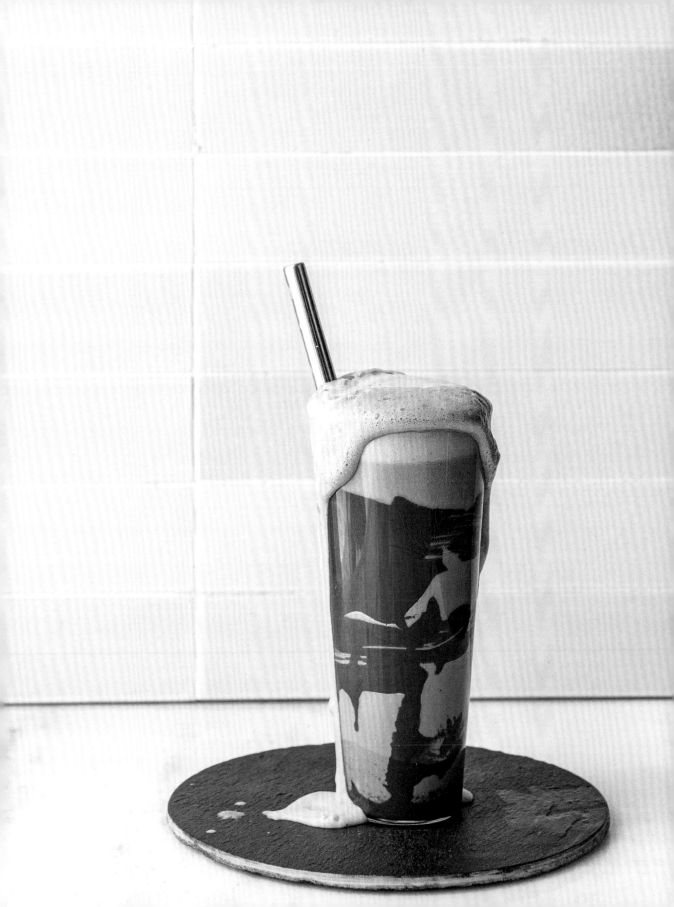

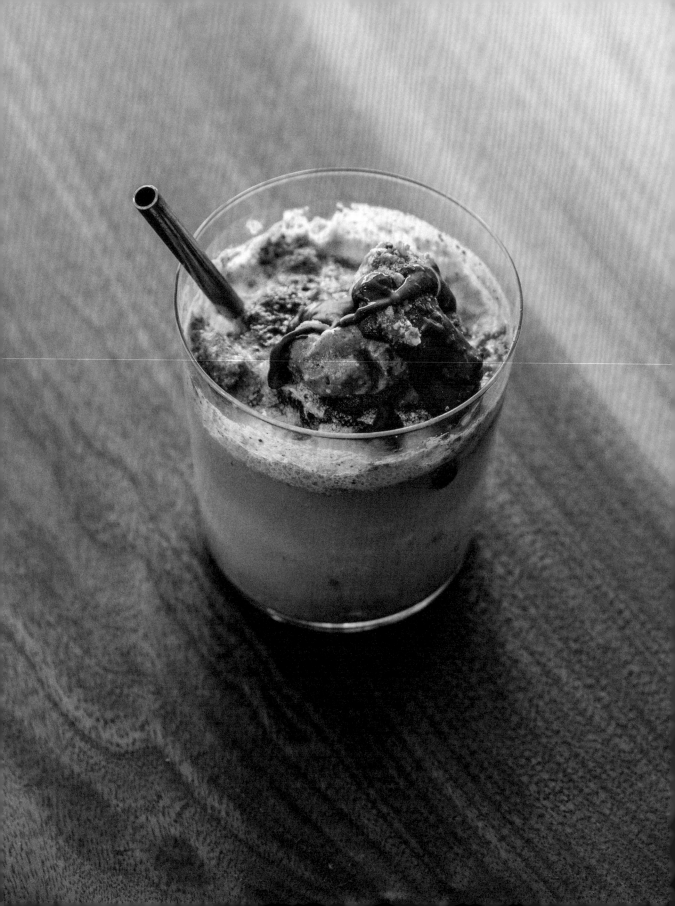

ashwagandha root tonic

Ashwagandha is another adaptogen. It's been shown to lower blood sugar levels, reduce cortisol, help brain function, and combat signs of anxiety and depression. Needless to say, I use it a lot and it's very complementary to CBD. I find it particularly useful in the evenings, just before bed, which is why this recipe works like a decadent bedtime snack.

—————— SERVES 2 ——————

4 ounces (95 g) dark vegan chocolate, coarsely chopped

2 tablespoons coconut butter (page 25) (or regular butter)

1 tablespoon maple syrup

½ cup (120 ml) nut milk (page 20 or 23)

½ teaspoon ground cinnamon

1 teaspoon ashwagandha root powder

30 milligrams CBD oil

16 ounces (480 ml) carbonated water

Hot fudge, caramel sauce (both on page 168), and store-bought freeze-dried strawberry powder, for serving (optional)

In a medium-size saucepan over low heat, melt the chocolate and coconut butter, stirring continuously (both burn easily, so be watchful). Once smooth, remove from the heat and stir in the maple syrup. Next, add the milk to the cooling pan, scraping down the sides with a rubber spatula. Transfer the concoction to a high-speed blender and add the cinnamon and ashwagandha root powder and blend on high for 1 to 2 minutes.

Decant the liquid into 2 glasses and dose each with 15 milligrams CBD oil. Divide the carbonated water between the glasses. Drizzle hot fudge and caramel sauce on top, and garnish with strawberry powder, if using. Drink immediately.

(GF)

(V)

apple and fennel sparkling "mocktail"

After you've been the "pregnant lady" for several years running you'll never look at cocktail parties the same way. I always make it a point to offer a nonalcoholic something, and CBD is a great additive because you can easily add it post-production for those who want it and omit it for those who don't. This one is delicious and always a crowd-pleaser.

—————————— SERVES 2 ——————————

FOR THE FENNEL SYRUP:

½ cup (65 grams) coconut sugar

1½ tablespoons fennel seeds (alternatively, use 1 fresh fennel bulb)

½ cup (120 ml) maple syrup

FOR THE MOCKTAIL:

8 ounces (240 ml) unsweetened apple juice

1 tablespoon fresh lemon juice

30 milligrams CBD oil

8 ounces (240 ml) carbonated water

Fennel fronds or apple wedges, for serving

Make the fennel syrup: In a medium saucepan over medium heat, bring ½ cup (120 ml) water, the coconut sugar, and fennel seeds to a boil. If using fresh fennel, cut a fennel bulb into large enough pieces for easy removal but small enough to be submerged in the liquid, about the size of a thumb. Continue to cook over medium heat, stirring every few minutes to ensure the mixture doesn't run dry or scorch, for 20 minutes or until a rich, combined, dark brown.

Remove from the heat and discard the seeds, or large chunks of fennel, by pouring through a fine-mesh sieve or nut milk bag. Stir in the maple syrup.

Make the mocktail: Fill each glass or mason jar with ½ cup (120 ml) ice. Divide the apple juice between jars, followed by lemon juice, fennel syrup, CBD oil, and finally, carbonated water. Garnish with fennel fronds or apple wedges and drink immediately.

GF

V

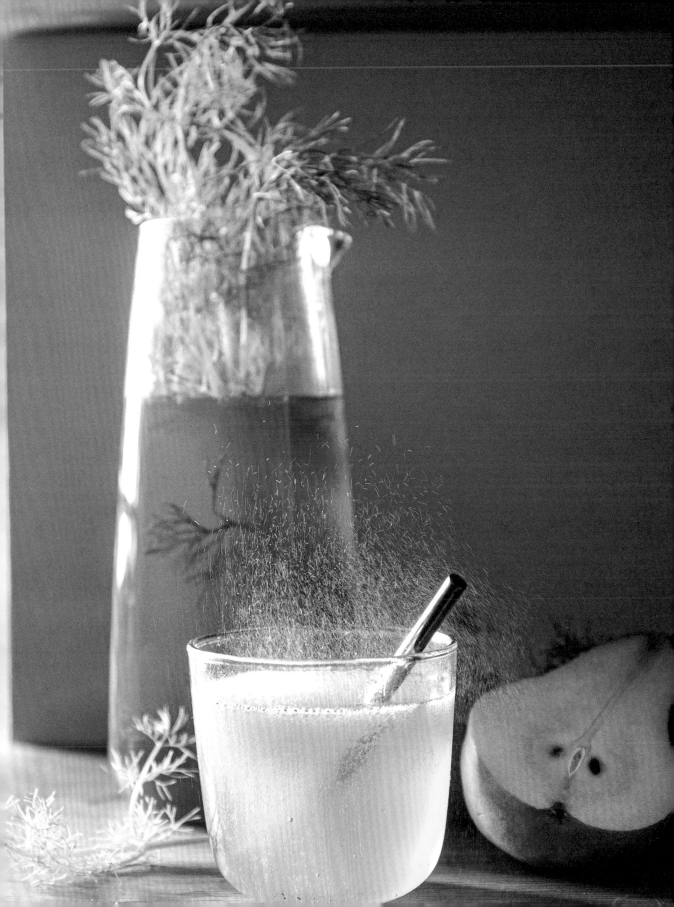

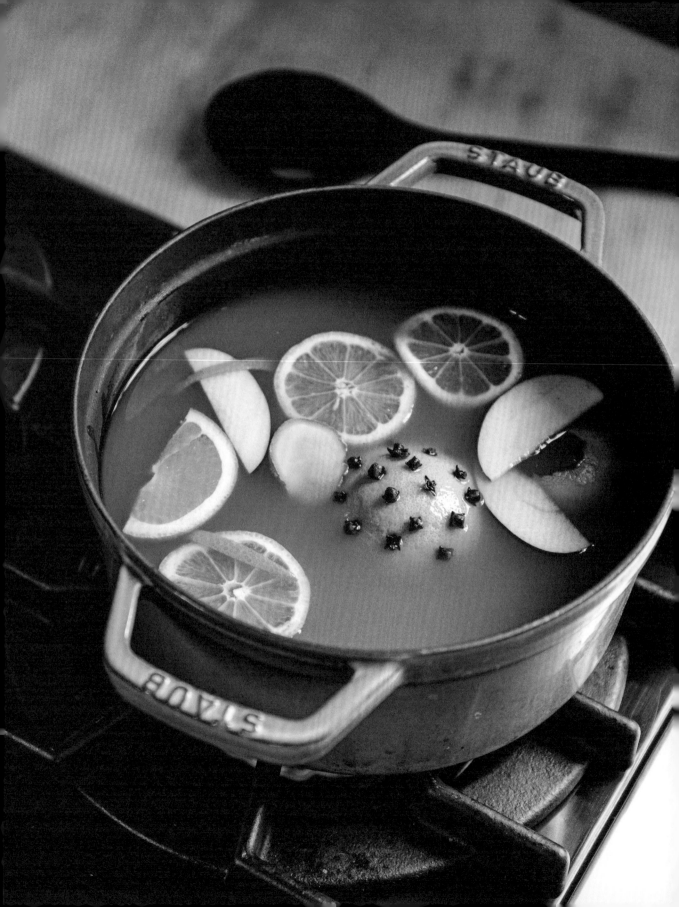

"spiked" apple cider

I'm not talking spiked with alcohol but instead CBD. While I'm a huge fan of the entire holiday season (it drives my husband crazy—the day after Halloween I'm cueing up Nat King Cole's holiday catalog), I drink this spiced cider year-round, hot and cold, because it's easy to make, delicious, filled with antioxidants, and makes the whole house smell amazing.

——————————— SERVES 2 ———————————

1 cinnamon stick, crushed

½ teaspoon whole cloves

½ teaspoon whole black peppercorns

1 teaspoon ground nutmeg

1 orange, zested

16 ounces (480 ml) unsweetened apple juice

30 milligrams CBD oil

In a Dutch oven or large saucepan over medium heat, dry roast the cinnamon stick, cloves, and peppercorns until aromatic, for 1 to 2 minutes. Add the nutmeg and roast for about a minute more before adding the orange zest and apple juice. Heat the mixture at medium for 10 to 12 minutes, until mixture comes to a rolling boil, then reduce heat to medium low and simmer for another 20 to 30 minutes. Pour the cider through a fine-mesh sieve or nut milk bag to remove the whole spices.

Decant into mugs and dose each serving with 15 milligrams CBD oil. Enjoy.

GF

V

sweet alice apple kombucha

My daughter is an Alice, and when we happened to find the Sweet Alice variety of apples we made it a point to use them for pretty much everything involving apples. Trader Joe's sells them when they're in season, as do many farmers' markets.

———————————— SERVES 2 ————————————

1 pound (500 g) or about 3 Sweet Alice apples (any nice, sweet red apple like Gala or Honeycrisp will do if you have a juicer; or use ½ cup [120 ml] store-bought unsweetened apple juice)

¼ teaspoon ground ginger

1 lemon, zested and juiced

16 ounces (480 ml) plain kombucha*

30 milligrams CBD oil

If you are using fresh apples, run them through a juicer.

In a pitcher or jar, stir together the apple juice, ginger, and lemon juice; add the kombucha. Mix well and divide between 2 pint glasses or mason jars before dosing each with 15 milligrams CBD oil.

*You can swap in tea or carbonated water for the kombucha.

ginger lime kombucha

This is my favorite kombucha for summer—it's dangerously easy to drink and perfect on a hot day. For something lighter, the ginger-lime syrup is also delicious topped off with caronated water. I strongly encourage fresh ginger for this one.

───────── SERVES 2 ─────────

½ cup (65 grams) coconut sugar

1 small knuckle-size piece of ginger (about 2 to 4 ounces), peeled

¼ cup (60 ml) fresh lime juice (from about 2 to 3 limes)

16 ounces (480 ml) plain kombucha

30 milligrams CBD oil

In a small saucepan, combine the coconut sugar, ginger, and lime juice with ½ cup (120 ml) water and bring to a boil over high heat until the sugar is fully dissolved, about 10 minutes. Remove from the heat and discard the piece of ginger. Refrigerate until cool (2 to 4 hours) before adding to the kombucha in a large pitcher; stir to combine.

Decant into 2 glasses and dose each with 15 milligrams CBD oil.

GF

V

lavender lemon kombucha

I was never much of a lavender person until moving to Los Angeles. Here it grows almost effortlessly on the hillsides, pouring over garden walls and just waiting to be used for something. Then I started making a simple lavender syrup, and once I got that down I began adding it to everything.

SERVES 2

½ cup (65 grams) coconut sugar

1 tablespoon culinary-grade dried lavender blossoms

½ cup (120 ml) fresh lemon juice

16 ounces (480 ml) plain kombucha

30 milligrams CBD oil

Fresh lavender or mint leaves, for serving (optional)

In a small saucepan over high heat, heat the coconut sugar with ½ cup (120 ml) of water along with the dried lavender and lemon juice to make the simple syrup. Bring to a boil, then simmer for 15 to 20 minutes before removing from the heat and allowing the mixture to cool. Once cooled, pour through a fine-mesh sieve or nut milk bag to remove the lavender blossoms; refrigerate for 2 to 4 hours.

Pour the syrup and kombucha into a large pitcher and stir before decanting into 2 pint glasses or mason jars and dosing each with 15 milligrams CBD oil. Garnish with fresh lavender or mint if you want it to be a little fancy.

GF

V

grapefruit and thyme kombucha

We have a grapefruit tree alongside a community staircase in our neighborhood that's part of my running route. Every year it bursts into magnificent, floral- and citrus-scented orbs and I gather them in my shirt and run home looking pretty crazy. This is my favorite thing to do with them.

──── SERVES 2 ────

¼ cup (60 ml) fresh grapefruit juice

½ cup (65 grams) coconut sugar

5 to 10 fresh sprigs of thyme, plus more for serving (optional)

16 ounces (480 ml) plain kombucha

30 milligrams CBD oil

Grapefruit wedges, for serving (optional)

In a small saucepan over high heat, heat the grapefruit juice, coconut sugar, thyme sprigs, and about ¼ cup (60 ml) of water to make the simple syrup. Bring to a boil, then simmer for 15 to 20 minutes before removing from the heat and allowing the mixture to cool. Once cooled, pour it through a fine-mesh sieve or nut milk bag to remove the thyme bits; refrigerate for 2 to 4 hours.

Pour the syrup and kombucha into a large pitcher and stir well. Decant into 2 pint glasses or mason jars and dose each with 15 milligrams CBD oil. Garnish with thyme sprigs or grapefruit wedges (or both).

GF

V

almond butter and spinach smoothie

In my experience this is the most congenial of all smoothies: Everyone likes it. It's also a great way to use up kale stems or old greens about to miss their prime. Throw them in the freezer and use them for smoothies.

— SERVES 2 —

2 cups (480 ml) cashew or almond milk (page 20 or 23; store-bought will also work)

1 cup (30 g) fresh spinach, or a handful of frozen kale stems

2 frozen bananas

2 dates, pitted

2 heaping tablespoons almond butter (any nut butter will do)

½ teaspoon pure vanilla extract

¼ teaspoon ground cinnamon

½ cup (75 g) ice

30 milligrams CBD oil

Caramel sauce (page 168) and toasted almond slices, for serving (optional)

In a high-speed blender, combine spinach, bananas, dates, almond butter, vanilla, cinnamon and ice (everything but the CBD) and blend on high until smooth and creamy, 2 to 3 minutes. Divide evenly into 2 glasses and dose each with 15 milligrams CBD oil. Stir well and add a straw if you'd like. If you want a dessert, swirl your glass and top your smoothie with some vegan caramel sauce and sprinkle with toasted almond slices.

GF

V

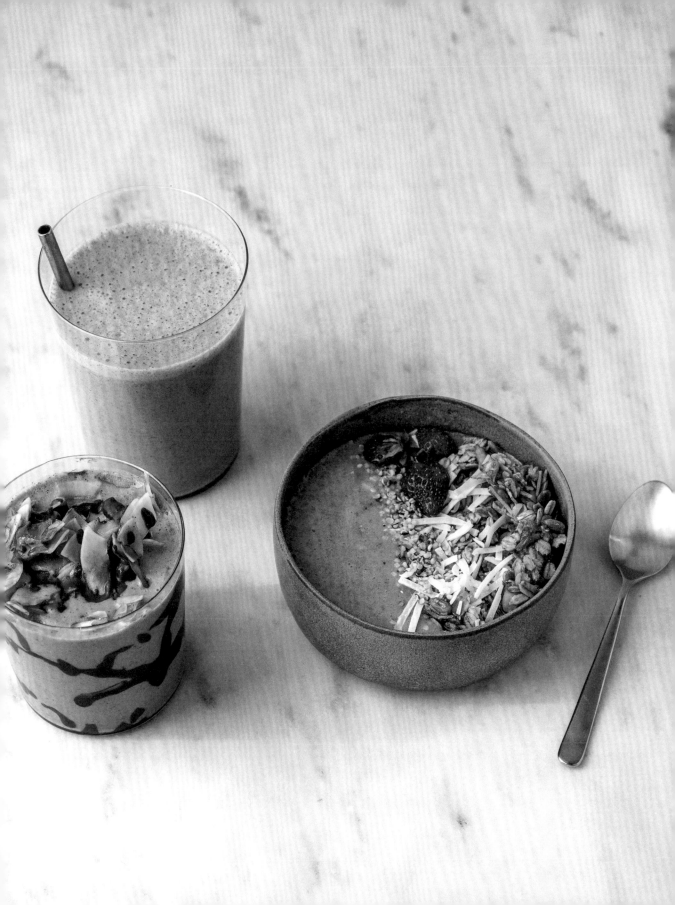

elvis smoothie

When I mentioned smoothies as desserts I specifically meant *this* smoothie. I like Elvis as much as the next person, but I love peanut butter, and my eye is now trained to scan menus for his name—pancakes, pie, etc.—because it's a clear indication peanut butter and something salty will be involved.

——————————— SERVES 2 ———————————

2 cups (480 ml) cashew or almond milk (page 20 or 23; or use store-bought nut milk)

2 frozen bananas

2 heaping tablespoons peanut butter

1 tablespoon maple syrup

½ tablespoon cocoa powder

½ cup (75 g) ice

30 milligrams CBD oil

Hot fudge (page 168) and coconut bacon (page 171), for serving (optional)

In a high-speed blender, combine nut milk, bananas, peanut butter, syrup, and cocoa powder with ½ cup ice and blend for 2 to 3 minutes, until all ingredients are fully combined. Divide evenly between 2 glasses and dose each with 15 milligrams CBD oil.

If you really want to go full-on dessert, I strongly encourage both hot fudge and coconut bacon. Just don't forget to omit the CBD oil from the sauce unless you'd like a double dose!

Picture page 67.

GF

V

strawberry banana smoothie

I studied abroad for a year in college and my roommate would eat neither strawberries nor bananas because she had apparently *only* eaten them for most of her babyhood and childhood. I can't imagine ever growing tired of the combination, which is why this smoothie remains my favorite.

———————————————— SERVES 2 ————————————————

2 cups (290 grams) frozen strawberries

2 frozen bananas

2 cups (480 ml) cashew or almond milk (page 20 or 23; or use store-bought nut milk)

1 tablespoon maple syrup

1 teaspoon pure vanilla extract

30 milligrams CBD oil

Granola (page 75), fresh strawberries, coconut flakes, and hemp seeds, for serving (optional)

In a high-speed blender, combine frozen strawberries, bananas, nut milk, maple syrup, and vanilla (all ingredients except the CBD) and blend on high until smooth, 2 to 3 minutes. Divide evenly between 2 bowls and dose each with 15 milligrams CBD oil.

For a crunchy finish, top with granola (just don't forget to omit the CBD from the recipe unless you want a double dose!) and layer with fresh strawberries, coconut flakes, and hemp seeds.

Picture page 67.

GF

V

breakfast

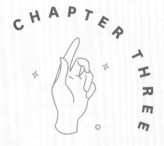

CHAPTER THREE

peanut butter and chocolate overnight oats

Meal prep can be a beautiful thing, and overnight oats are fairly genius. Making them in a jar helps keep them very portable, too, so they can be enjoyed anywhere. In my opinion this is the only kind of overnight oats worth eating. Granted, I have a preoccupation with peanut butter, but this recipe is so insanely good I have a hard time eating anything else when this is available to me.

SERVES 1

2½ tablespoons peanut butter

¼ teaspoon pure vanilla extract

Pinch of sea salt

½ tablespoon maple syrup

½ tablespoon cocoa powder

¼ cup (25 g) gluten-free rolled oats

¼ cup (55 g) coconut or cashew yogurt (page 26; store-bought will also work)

¼ cup (60 ml) nut milk (page 20 or 23)

15 milligrams CBD oil

Chocolate chips (optional)

In a small saucepan over low heat, gently heat the peanut butter, vanilla, salt, and maple syrup, stirring constantly, until smooth and combined. Add the cocoa powder and stir until incorporated and then stir in the oats. Remove from the heat and add yogurt, milk, and CBD oil, stirring together before putting the mixture in a 16-ounce (480 ml) mason jar with a lid. Top the mixture with chocolate chips if you want to make it a dessert—it's outstanding. Refrigerate overnight or for up to 5 days.

GF

V

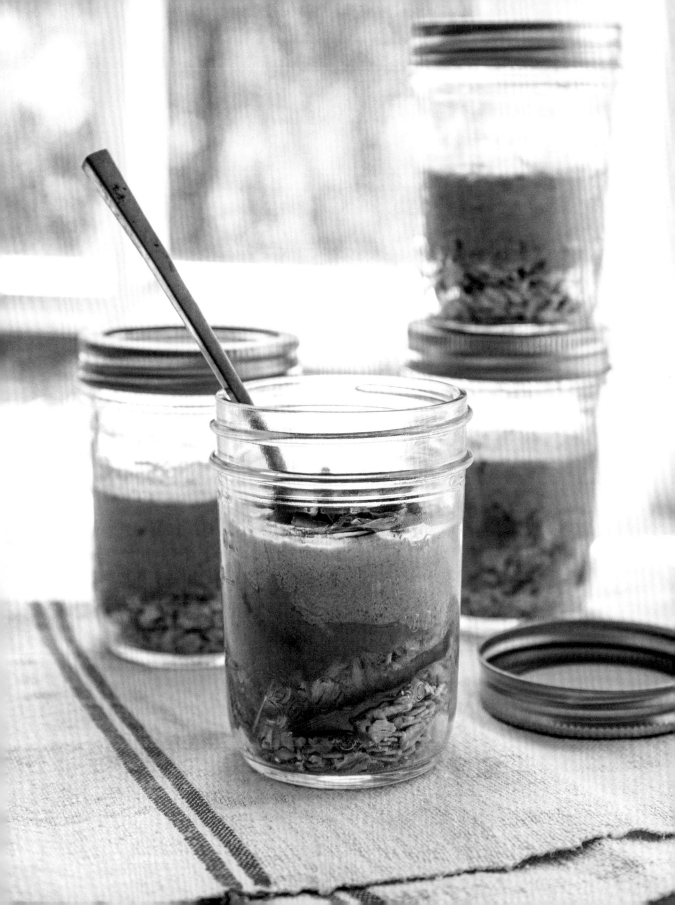

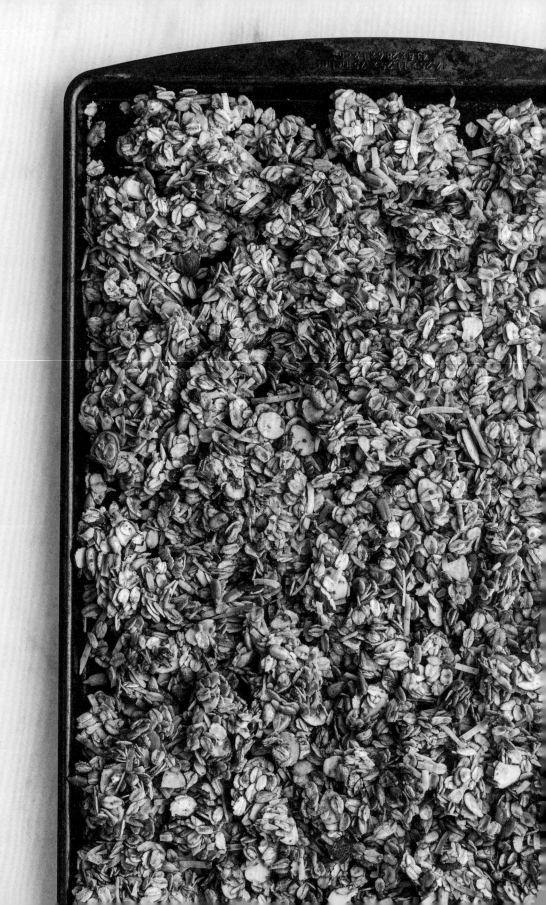

granola

Next to peanut butter, I really love granola. I even eat it on ice cream. There's just nothing with a crunch factor that I prefer more (except maybe crème brûlée). This is my favorite granola because it's chunky and can almost stand in for a healthy-ish cookie.

—————— **MAKES ABOUT 20 (½-CUP / 65 G) SERVINGS** ——————

5 cups (450 g) gluten-free rolled oats

1 cup (100 g) dried coconut flakes

1 cup (125 g) sunflower seeds

1 cup (150 g) sliced raw almonds

½ teaspoon sea salt

½ cup (95 g) coconut oil

½ cup (120 ml) maple syrup

⅓ cup (25 g) coconut sugar

1 tablespoon pure vanilla extract

300 milligrams CBD oil*

Preheat the oven to 350° F (180° C). Line 2 baking sheets with parchment paper.

In the bowl of a stand mixer or large, heavy-bottomed bowl, combine the oats, coconut flakes, sunflower seeds, almonds, and salt; run mixer on low (or stir well) until the ingredients are fully incorporated, about 1 minute. In a small saucepan over low heat, melt the coconut oil until it has turned to liquid; remove from the heat. Add the maple syrup, coconut sugar, vanilla, and CBD oil to the same pan. Pour the wet ingredients into the dry ingredients a bit at a time, making sure everything is fully mixed and saturated.

Distribute the granola evenly across both parchment-lined baking sheets.

Bake for 6 to 7 minutes, then rotate the sheets to different shelves to ensure even baking. Stir up any darker oats, etc., then cook for another 6 to 7 minutes. A great clue to doneness is when you start to smell granola—it burns quickly, so don't forget it! Allow oats to cool fully before handling so the CBD oil will dry and the granola can properly clump.

If you plan to use the granola as a base for vegan granola bars, omit the CBD and use the measurements for Baked Granola Bars (page 100) instead.

GF

V

apple fritter pancake bites

I don't care about any donut except apple fritters. I've been this way my entire life. As a kid, I spent my Saturdays eating Dunkin' Donuts apple fritters with a mini-carton of chocolate milk served with a straw in a scratched-up glass—I thought it was heaven on earth. These are much better for you, which means a lot to me now that I'm an adult and focused on eating healthful foods!

SERVES 7 (2 FRITTERS PER PERSON)

FOR THE FRITTERS:

1 cup (130 g) coconut sugar, divided

1 tablespoon ground cinnamon

½ cup (65 g) blanched almond flour

1½ cups (180 g) all-purpose flour

¼ teaspoon sea salt

1½ teaspoons baking powder

1 egg

1 cup (240 ml) applesauce

⅔ cup (125 g) coconut oil or avocado oil for frying

FOR THE GLAZE:

1½ tablespoons almond milk (page 23), oat or cashew milk will work; too

2 tablespoons cultured vegan butter (page 28)

1 tablespoon maple syrup

1 teaspoon pure vanilla extract

1½ cups confectioner's sugar

105 milligrams CBD oil

Make the fritters: In a small bowl, whisk 2 tablespoons of the coconut sugar with the cinnamon and set aside. In a large bowl, mix the remaining dry ingredients: almond flour, all-purpose flour, what remains of the coconut sugar, as well as the salt and baking powder. Whisk to fully incorporate and add the coconut sugar and cinnamon mixture and whisk again. In a smaller bowl, stir together the egg and applesauce, mixing thoroughly. Add the wet and dry ingredients and blend by hand, loosely but vigorously, until there are no pockets of dry ingredients and everything is more or less smooth.

In a cast iron skillet or frying pan, heat the oil to around 370° F (190° C). Alternatively, heat the oil for 1 to 2 minutes until it crackles and curdles a test bit of dough, then set to medium heat to make sure it won't get too hot. Using a tablespoon, drop the donut hole–size bits of dough into the oil, browning on one side (about 30 to 45 seconds), before flipping to the other (they brown fast—watch them closely). Once both sides are golden, transfer to a baking sheet in a warm oven (300° F or 150° C) while you make remaining batches.

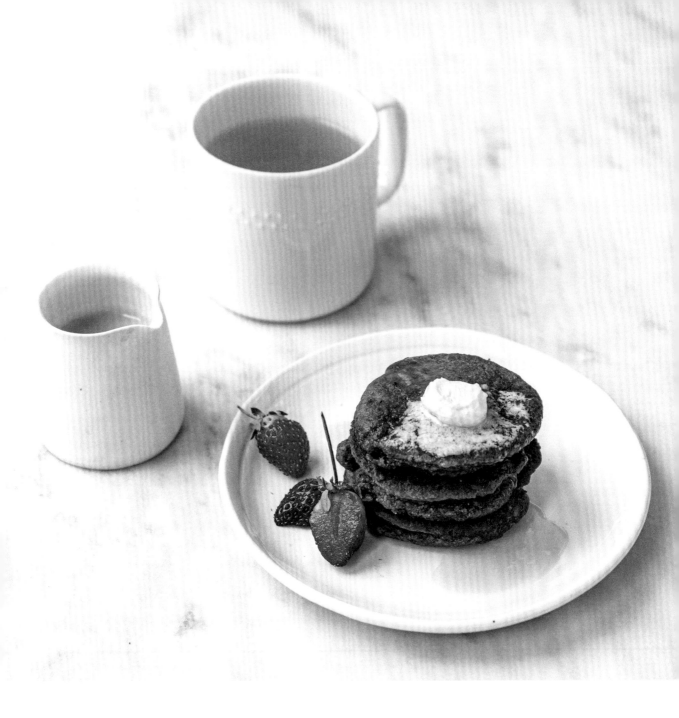

Make the glaze: In a small pan over medium heat, melt the cultured vegan butter into the almond milk, whisking continuously. Add the maple syrup, and vanilla, continuing to whisk until everything is incorporated, about 3 minutes. Once mixed, removed the pan from the heat and slowly stir in the confectioner's sugar a few tablespoons at a time. The glaze should be smooth, glassy, and creamy, and CBD can now be added.

Once the glaze is ready, remove the fritters from the oven and allow to cool for about 5 minutes before drizzling each pancake with the CBD glaze.

cinnamon rolls

This recipe uses dry yeast and is by far the most complicated in the book, but don't let that scare you! It's still easy and, like all these recipes, it's a slightly healthier take on something typically filled with junk ingredients. So worth it.

————————————— MAKES 12 ROLLS —————————————

FOR THE ROLLS:

1 cup (130 g) coconut sugar

1 packet of active dry yeast

3 cups (360 g) all-purpose flour, divided

1 cup (90 g) blanched almond flour

½ teaspoon sea salt

¼ cup (50 g) coconut oil, melted

FOR THE FILLING:

½ cup (65 g) coconut sugar

3 tablespoons coconut cream

2 tablespoons ground cinnamon

FOR THE ICING:

½ cup (100 g) cultured vegan butter (page 28), at room temperature

3 tablespoons coconut butter (page 25), at room temperature

¼ cup (30 g) confectioner's sugar

1 teaspoon pure vanilla extract

180 milligrams CBD oil

Make the dough: In a medium-size bowl, combine the coconut sugar, yeast, and 2 tablespoons of all-purpose flour with 1 cup (240 ml) of lukewarm water, whisking until the clumps are dissolved. Allow mixture to stand for 5 minutes. The mixture will begin to bubble and foam up a bit and smell like bread as it rises.

In the bowl of a stand mixer, combine the remaining flours with the salt; add the yeast mix. Using the hook attachment, mix the dough until it begins to come together loosely. When this happens, stop the mixer and add the coconut oil, then resume mixing, leaving the mixer to knead for 10 to 12 minutes.

Once the mixture had been kneaded into dough remove it from the bowl and transfer to a new, flour-dusted bowl and cover with a clean tea towel, allowing the dough to rise for at least an hour or two at room temperature.

Preheat the oven to 350° F (180° C). Line 2 baking sheets with parchment paper.

Make the filling: In a small bowl, mix together the coconut sugar, coconut cream, and cinnamon.

Assemble the rolls: Using a rolling pin (or a wine bottle) and your hands, roll out the dough into a large rectangle. It doesn't need to be precise, but 9 x 18 inches (22 x 45 cm) is ideal. Spread the filling across the flattened dough evenly and then, starting at one of the longer sides, roll the dough up into a long log.

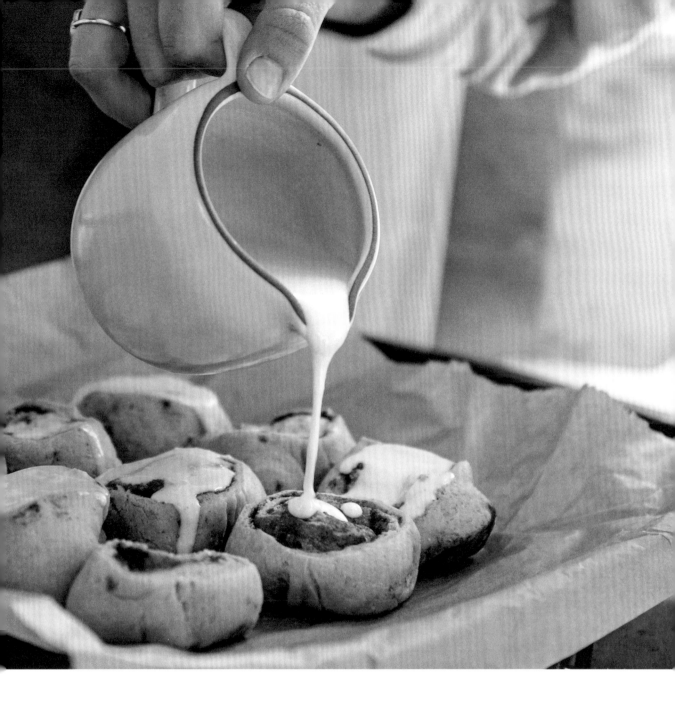

Using a knife, cut into 12 rolls and arrange them on the parchment-lined baking sheets. Bake the rolls until lightly browned on top, 17 to 20 minutes. Allow them to cool.

Meanwhile, make the icing: In a bowl, mix together the cultured butter, coconut butter, confectioner's sugar, vanilla, and CBD oil. Once the rolls are cool, ice each roll evenly.

These rolls are wonderful, but like many pastries, they don't store well. They're best eaten quickly, ideally the day they are made.

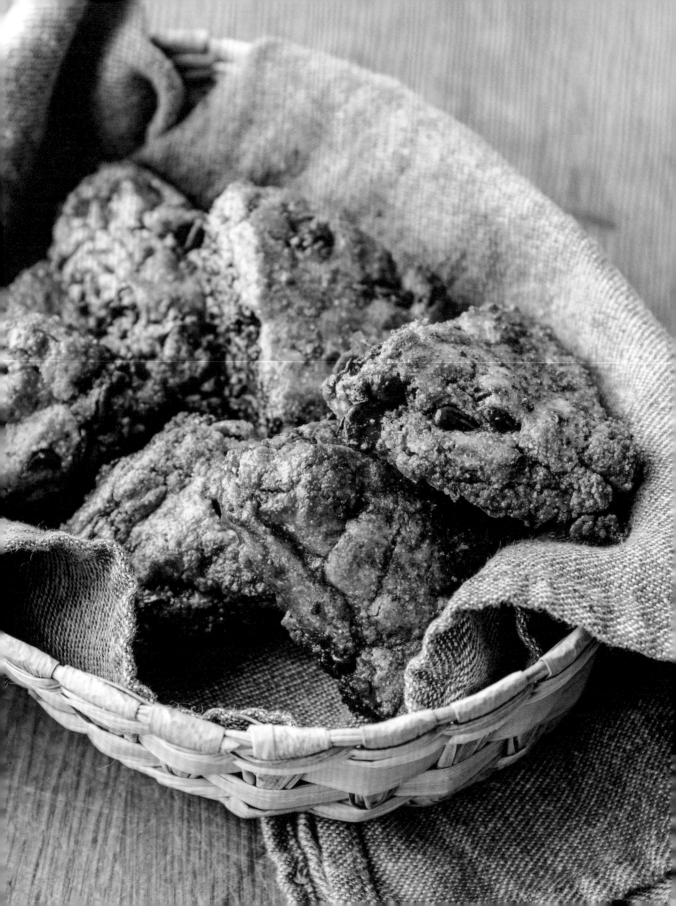

chocolate chip scones

I grew up thinking scones were something only found at a high tea. I've changed my mind and decided they're wonderfully rustic and the texture can't be beat—like sugared shortbread cookies.

—————————— MAKES 11 SCONES ——————————

1¼ cups (120 g) blanched almond flour (plus about 3½ tablespoons extra for rolling)

¼ cup (50 g) cultured vegan butter (page 28), melted

1½ tablespoons maple syrup

1 teaspoon pure vanilla extract

½ teaspoon sea salt

½ cup (65 g) coconut sugar (plus more for dusting prepped scones)

½ cup (90 g) chocolate chips

1 egg*

165 milligrams CBD oil

Preheat the oven to 350° F (180° C). Line a baking sheet with parchment paper.

In a medium-size bowl, combine the flour, melted vegan butter, maple syrup, vanilla, salt, and coconut sugar. Using your hands, loosely combine the ingredients, being careful not to overmix. When the dough is formed but still slightly floury, add the chocolate chips and turn out the dough onto a floured surface, shaping it into a long rectangle (like a train), about 10 to 12 inches (25 to 30 cm) pushing it tightly together.

Using a pastry knife (or a regular knife), cut the dough into diagonal wedges, creating triangle shapes and working through to the end.

Arrange the wedges on the parchment-lined baking sheet. In a small bowl, beat the egg. Using a pastry brush, lightly coat each wedge with the egg wash, sealing in the dough, followed by a scant handful of coconut sugar, before baking for 10 minutes. Check for browning edges and glossy, dried egg wash as a visual cue for doneness. Once you've removed them from the oven, dose each scone with 4 drops of CBD oil.

Scones can be kept up to 2 days in sealed container.

To make vegan, you can substitute 2 tablespoons aquafaba—the liquid in a can of chickpeas—for the egg.

GF

almond and pistachio pancakes

My daughter loves pancakes. In an effort to create a more filling, nutrient-dense pancake (without the addition of such offending things as zucchini or spinach!) I came up with these. They're delicious, and you won't be hungry again in an hour.

———— SERVES ABOUT 8 (2 PANCAKES PER SERVING) ————

¾ cup (90 g) all-purpose flour

¼ cup (20 g) almond flour

¼ cup (40 g) raw pistachios

½ teaspoon sea salt

2 eggs

1 cup (240 ml) nut milk (page 20 or 23)

2 tablespoons melted cultured vegan butter (page 28)

2 tablespoons coconut oil

120 milligrams CBD oil

Maple coconut butter (page 172), for serving (optional)

In a food processor or high-speed blender, process the flours, pistachios, and salt until they're ground into a coarse meal. Add the eggs, nut milk, and melted butter and process until just combined.

Heat the coconut oil in a heavy-bottomed skillet over medium heat. Drop about 2 tablespoons of batter per pancake, cooking each until it begins to bubble, then flip. Remove when golden-brown. Serve 2 pancakes per person, dosing each pancake with about 2 to 3 drops of oil immediately after cooking. These go great with the maple coconut butter, which can be heated in a small saucepan over medium heat and stirred continuously to avoid burning. Pour and serve immediately.

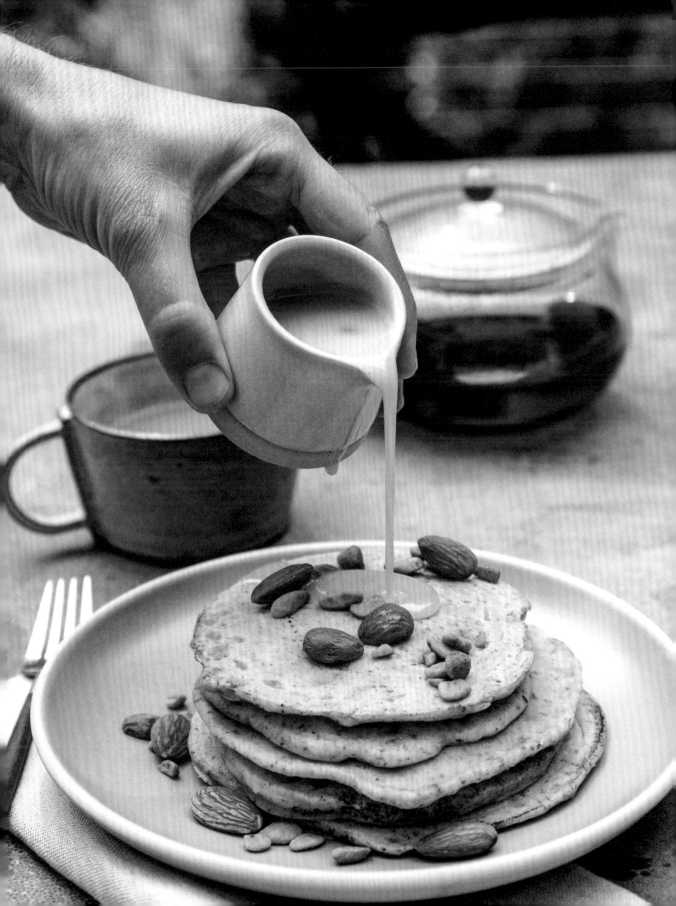

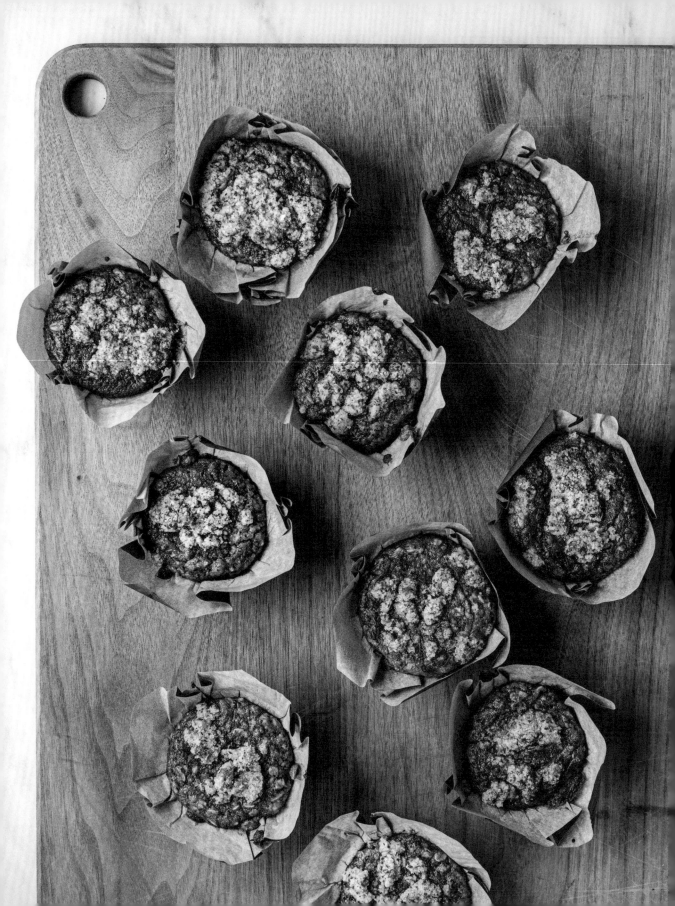

banana nut muffins

Bananas and walnuts are my favorite muffin combination, but this recipe is all about the topping. It turns out coconut sugar makes a rich and delicious type of crumble that's completely irresistible (and the rest of the muffin is delectable, too)!

——————————— **MAKES 17 MUFFINS** ———————————

2 tablespoons ground flaxseed

1 teaspoon pure vanilla extract

3 tablespoons coconut oil, melted

3 ripe bananas

¾ cup (180 ml) nut milk (page 20 or 23)

2 tablespoons maple syrup

⅓ cup (35 g) raw walnuts

1¼ cups (115 g) rolled oats

1½ cups (180 g) all-purpose flour

1 cup (80 g) almond flour

½ cup (65 g) coconut sugar

¼ teaspoon sea salt

1 teaspoon ground cinnamon

1 teaspoon baking powder

1 teaspoon baking soda

255 milligrams CBD oil

FOR THE TOPPING:

2 tablespoons coconut oil or cultured vegan butter (page 28)

⅓ cup (35 g) raw walnuts, chopped

½ cup (65 g) coconut sugar

2 tablespoons almond flour

Preheat the oven to 350° F (180° C). Line 17 muffin cups with paper baking cups.

In the bowl of a stand mixer or in a large bowl, combine the flaxseed with 2 tablespoons of warm water. Let this sit for a minute or two before adding the vanilla, coconut oil, and bananas. Mix on medium followed by high for 1 to 2 minutes, until the banana is mashed evenly into the batter (alternatively, you can mash and mix with your hands—it just takes a little longer). Stop the mixer and scrape down the sides of the bowl, then add nut milk, maple syrup, and walnuts—which will give them a chance to get chopped for you if you're using whole nuts; mix again for 1 minute.

In a separate bowl, whisk together the oats, both flours, sugar, salt, cinnamon, and baking powder and soda. Add the flour mixture to the stand mixer bowl and mix on low, moving up to high, for 2 minutes. Using a cookie scoop or large spoon, fill each muffin liner about three-quarters full. Top each muffin with about 4 drops (or 15 milligrams) of CBD oil.

Make the topping: In a small saucepan over low heat, melt the coconut oil or cultured vegan butter. Add the chopped walnuts followed by coconut sugar and almond flour to make a floury mixture—a crumble.

Top each muffin with a scant handful of topping and bake until a toothpick inserted in the center comes out clean, 35 to 40 minutes, or until the toppings have browned and the muffins are fragrant.

(V)

blueberry muffins

I always have blueberry muffins on Mondays, mostly because Mondays are hard, and CBD and a warm muffin make almost anything seem possible.

———— MAKES 12 MUFFINS ————

½ cup (100 g) cultured vegan butter (page 28)

1½ tablespoons ground flaxseed

1 ripe banana

¾ cup (120 g) coconut sugar

¾ cup (180 ml) almond milk (page 23)

2 tablespoons fresh lemon juice

1 teaspoons pure vanilla extract

1 cup (120 g) all-purpose flour

1 cup (80 g) almond flour

1 teaspoon baking powder

¼ teaspoon baking soda

¼ teaspoon sea salt

1 cup fresh blueberries

180 milligrams CBD oil

Preheat the oven to 350° F (180° C). Line 12 muffin cups with paper baking cups.

In a small saucepan, melt and brown the vegan butter, watching it to make sure it doesn't burn. In the bowl of a stand mixer or in a large bowl, combine the flaxseed with 2 tablespoons warm water; allow to sit for 1 to 2 minutes. Add the browned vegan butter along with the banana, coconut sugar, almond milk, lemon juice, and vanilla, mixing until smooth but not overbeaten, 1 to 2 minutes.

In a separate bowl, whisk together the all-purpose flour, almond flour, baking powder, baking soda, and salt. Add the dry ingredients to the wet ingredients, a cup at a time, mixing until the batter is smooth (though it may still be lumpy). Fold in blueberries gently. Spoon around 2 tablespoons of batter into each muffin liner so they're three-quarters full, to avoid overflow. Top each muffin with about 4 drops (or 15 milligrams) CBD oil.

Bake until muffin tops turn golden and springy, or a toothpick inserted in the center comes out clean, about 17 to 20 minutes. Cool for 15 to 20 minutes before eating.

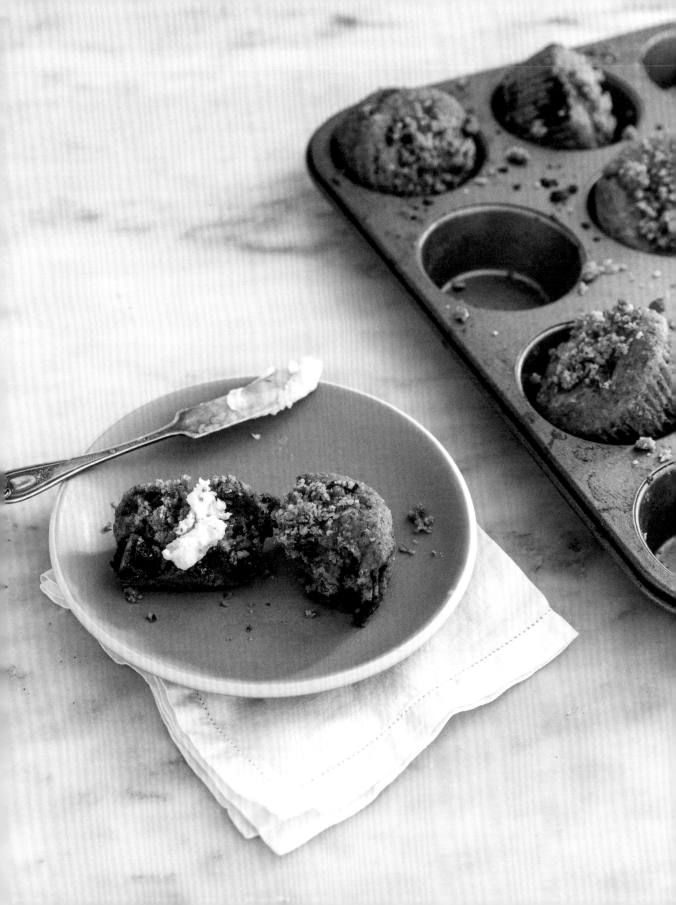

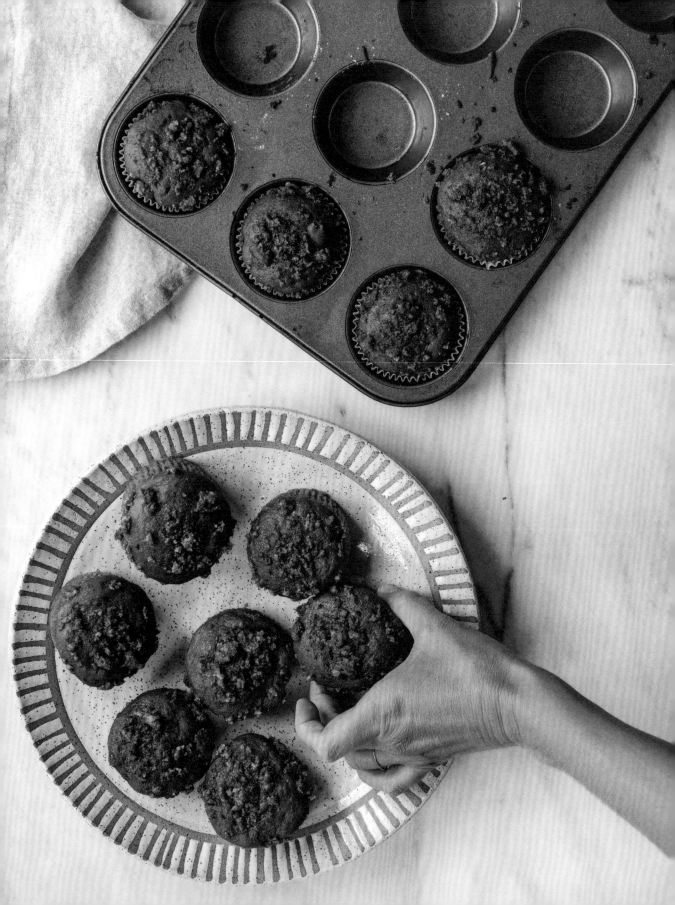

pumpkin apple muffins

I wouldn't have thought pumpkin-and-apple would be such a big thing until I made these. They're like fall in a muffin liner, with CBD.

───────── MAKES 18 MUFFINS ─────────

FOR THE MUFFINS:
2½ cups (300 g) all-purpose flour

2 cups (260 g) coconut sugar

1 teaspoon ground cinnamon

1 teaspoon ground ginger

½ teaspoon ground nutmeg

1 teaspoon baking soda

½ teaspoon sea salt

2 eggs

1 cup (225 g) pumpkin puree

½ cup (120 ml) olive oil

½ cup (120 g) applesauce

270 milligrams CBD oil

FOR THE STREUSEL:
3 tablespoons all-purpose flour

¼ cup (35 g) coconut sugar

½ teaspoon ground cinnamon

2 tablespoons cultured vegan butter (page 28)

Preheat the oven to 350° F (or 180° C). Line 18 muffin cups with paper baking cups. Oil paper baking cups (for insurance and easy release).

Make the muffins: In the bowl of a stand mixer or in a large bowl, mix together the flour, coconut sugar, spices, baking soda, and salt. In a separate bowl, whisk the eggs, then whisk in the pumpkin puree and olive oil; add into the dry ingredients, mixing just until moist. Add the applesauce and fold in gently, filling each muffin liner three-quarters full. Top each muffin with 4 drops of CBD oil (or 15 milligrams).

Make the streusel: In a small bowl, combine the flour, coconut sugar, and cinnamon. Melt the vegan butter in a small saucepan and pour it over the dry ingredients, using fingers to make a crumble. Distribute the crumble evenly over each muffin and bake until the tops have browned and a toothpick inserted in the center comes out clean, 12 to 15 minutes.

snacks & small treats

peanut butter energy bites

Flax is high in omega-3 fatty acids and it's a high-quality protein. It's pretty much the perfect ingredient in a midday treat.

───────── MAKES 15 BITES ─────────

¾ cup (195 g) peanut butter

2 tablespoons maple syrup

1 cup (90 g) gluten-free rolled oats

½ cup (60 g) ground flaxseed

½ cup (90 g) chocolate chips

225 milligrams CBD oil

In a small saucepan over low heat, gently heat the peanut butter and maple syrup, stirring until smooth. Remove from the heat and add the oats and ground flaxseed, stirring into a thick batter. Once cooled slightly, fold in the chocolate chips.

On a sheet of parchment paper, measure a heaping tablespoon of dough and roll between your hands into a ball. Repeat to make 15 balls and carefully dose each ball with 15 milligrams CBD oil (the oats will help absorb the oil and keep it from pooling). Allow the balls to sit in the fridge or freezer for about 30 minutes to an hour before eating.

GF

V

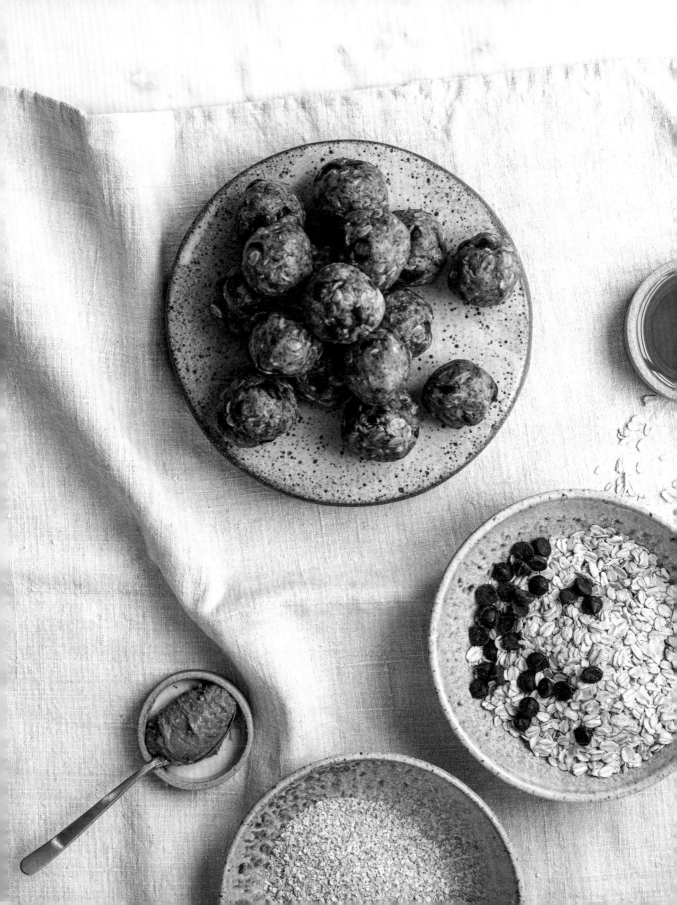

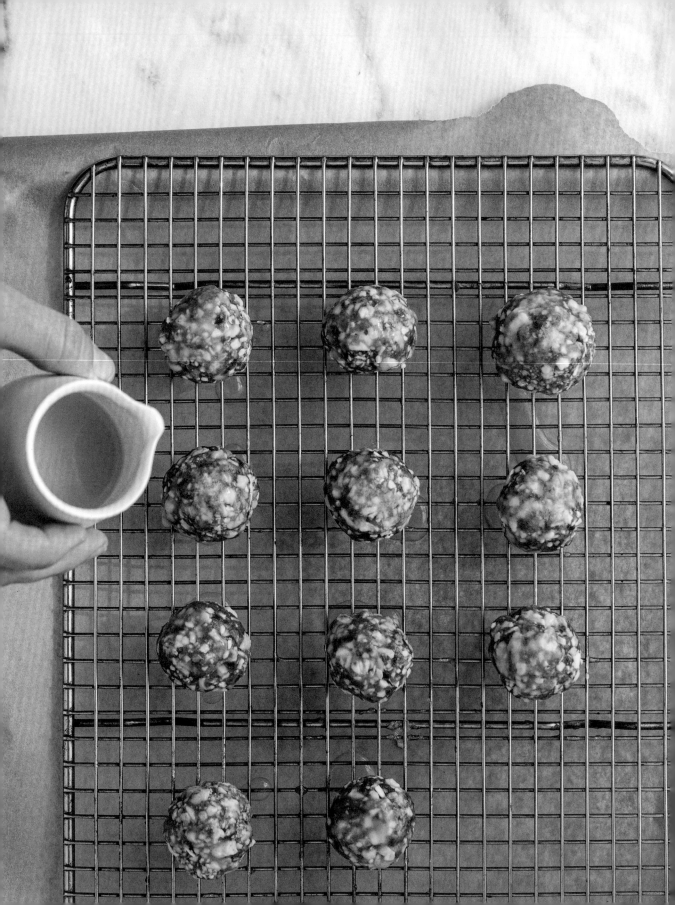

"donut holes"

I use quotations because these are not technically donut holes, but there are some satisfying similarities, so let's just go with it.

———————————— MAKES 12 DONUT HOLES ————————————

FOR THE DONUT HOLES:

1 cup (150 g) raw cashews

⅔ cup (65 g) shredded coconut flakes

8 dates, pitted

1 teaspoon pure vanilla extract

¼ teaspoon sea salt

180 milligrams CBD oil

FOR THE GLAZE:

1 tablespoon maple syrup

1 tablespoon coconut butter (page 25)

1 tablespoon coconut sugar

Make the donut holes: In a food processor, blend the cashews, shredded coconut, dates, vanilla, and salt until the mixture begins to form a large ball, about 1 or 2 minutes. For each donut hole, use a tablespoon to scoop a heaping spoonful and use your hands to make a round ball. Repeat to make 12 balls, setting each on a sheet of parchment paper.

Using a fork or a toothpick, make a small hole in the top of each ball and dose each with 15 milligrams CBD oil (the small repository will keep the oil inside the treat).

Make the glaze: In a small saucepan over low heat, warm the coconut butter and maple syrup, stirring continuously until fully melted and incorporated. Pour over the balls and let harden at room temperature.

On a plate, sprinkle the tablespoon of coconut sugar and roll each ball through it, creating a scant dusting for each treat.

GF

V

date and tahini caramels

These are a grown-up take on caramels, using healthful options for more complex flavors that taste delicious and will make you feel good.

———————————— **MAKES ABOUT 24 CARAMELS** ————————————

8 dates, pitted

2 tablespoons gluten-free tahini

¼ teaspoon sea salt, plus more for sprinkling

1 tablespoon maple syrup

360 milligrams CBD oil

2 ounces (55 g) dark chocolate (optional)

1 tablespoon coconut butter, melted (page 25; optional)

In a high-speed blender or food processor, combine the dates, tahini, salt, and maple syrup and blend until smooth and thick. Pour mixture into 24 mini-cupcake cups, filling about three-quarters full. Dose each with 15 milligrams CBD oil and sprinkle with salt.

Freeze for 2 to 4 hours, and keep cool until ready to eat.

Optionally, you can dip the caramels in a dark chocolate coating after solidly freezing the caramels for at least 4 hours. After melting the dark chocolate, combine it with the coconut butter, and dip the caramels one by one.

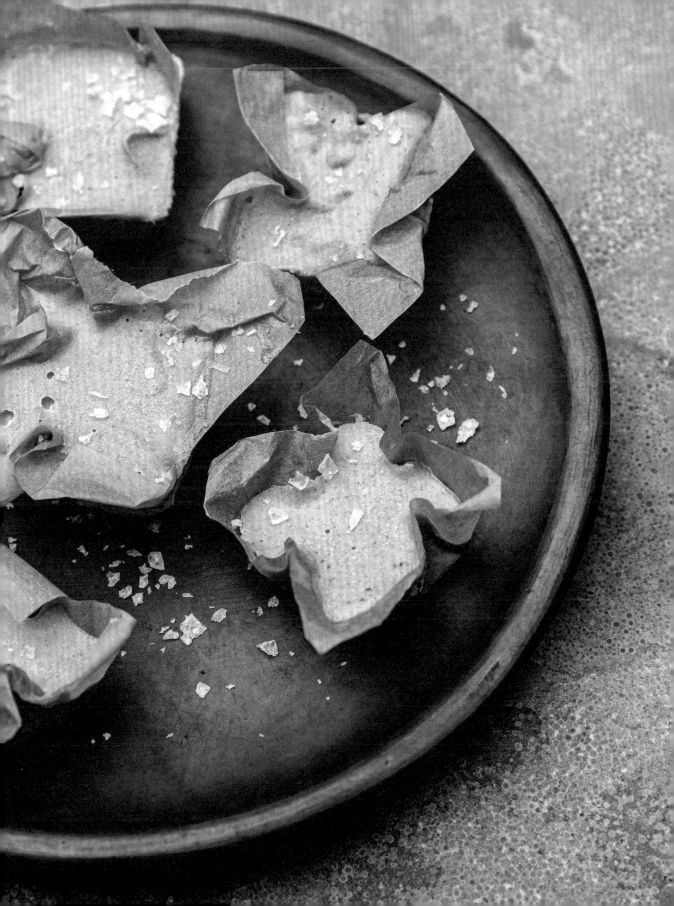

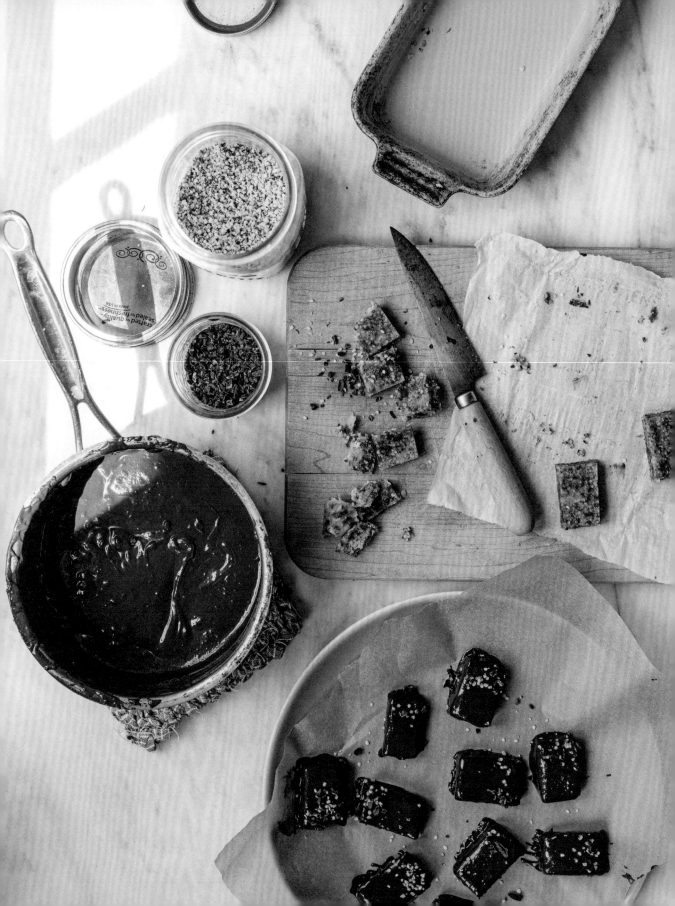

coconut butter hemp seed chocolate bites

These one-bite treats look beautiful despite their overall simplicity. They come out looking incredibly polished, but don't require any bake time (don't tell anyone!). They're also terribly hardy once constructed, safe inside a chocolate casing.

─────────── MAKES 12 BITES ───────────

FOR THE FILLING:
½ cup (120 ml) maple syrup

2 tablespoons coconut butter (page 25)

1 teaspoon pure vanilla extract

1 cup (160 g) hemp seeds

¼ teaspoon sea salt

180 milligrams CBD oil

FOR THE CHOCOLATE COATING:
1 cup (180 g) chocolate chips

2 tablespoons coconut butter (page 25)

Line a 5 x 7-inch (13 x 18-cm) mini rectangular baking pan with parchment paper.

Make the filling: In a small saucepan over low heat, combine the maple syrup and coconut butter, stirring continuously. Add the vanilla and remove from the heat. Stir in the hemp seeds and salt to make a dough. Add the CBD oil and knead with a metal spoon, stirring and fully incorporating the oil.

Press the dough flatly and evenly in the parchment-lined pan* (use an additional sheet of parchment to cover your hand so as not to disturb the oil). Freeze for 30 minutes to an hour before cutting the dough into small, 1 x 1-inch (2.5 x 2.5-cm) squares.

Make the chocolate coating: In a small saucepan over low heat, melt the chocolate chips with the coconut butter, stirring constantly. Once warm and smooth, remove from the heat.

Using a fork, run the hemp squares through the chocolate, lightly coating them. Use the rim of the pan to remove excess chocolate before gently pushing the now chocolate-covered pieces onto the parchment paper. Transfer the chocolates to the freezer or fridge to let cool for half an hour. Keep cool until ready to eat.

Alternatively, you can make teaspoon-size balls.

GF

V

baked granola bars

These amazing bars are made using my granola recipe and an egg with a few yummy bells and whistles.

———————————————— MAKES 6 BARS ————————————————

1½ cups (200 g) granola (page 75)

2 tablespoons peanut butter

½ cup (90 g) chocolate chips

1 egg, beaten to blend

1 teaspoon pure vanilla extract

90 milligrams CBD oil

Preheat the oven to 350° F (180° C). Line a 5 x 7-inch (13 x 18-cm) mini rectangular baking pan with parchment paper.

In a bowl, combine the granola with the peanut butter and the chocolate chips. Stir well, then add the egg and vanilla. Mix until the mixture is damp before turning out into the parchment-lined pan. Using clean hands or another sheet of parchment, press the mixture firmly into the pan. Bake until golden brown, 6 to 8 minutes. Remove from the oven then gently score the lines of your bars before dosing each with 15 milligrams CBD oil.

GF

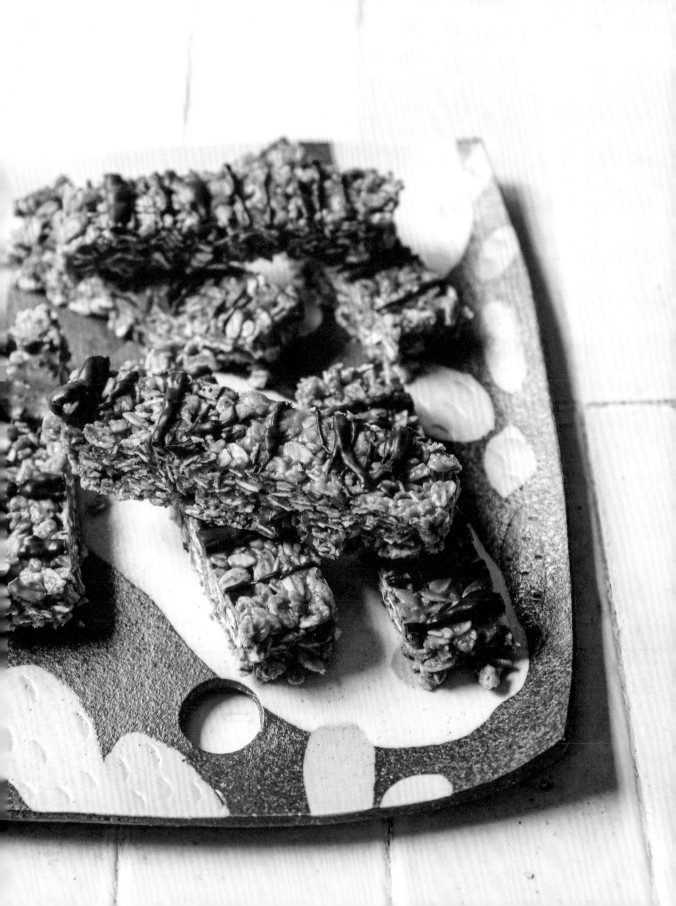

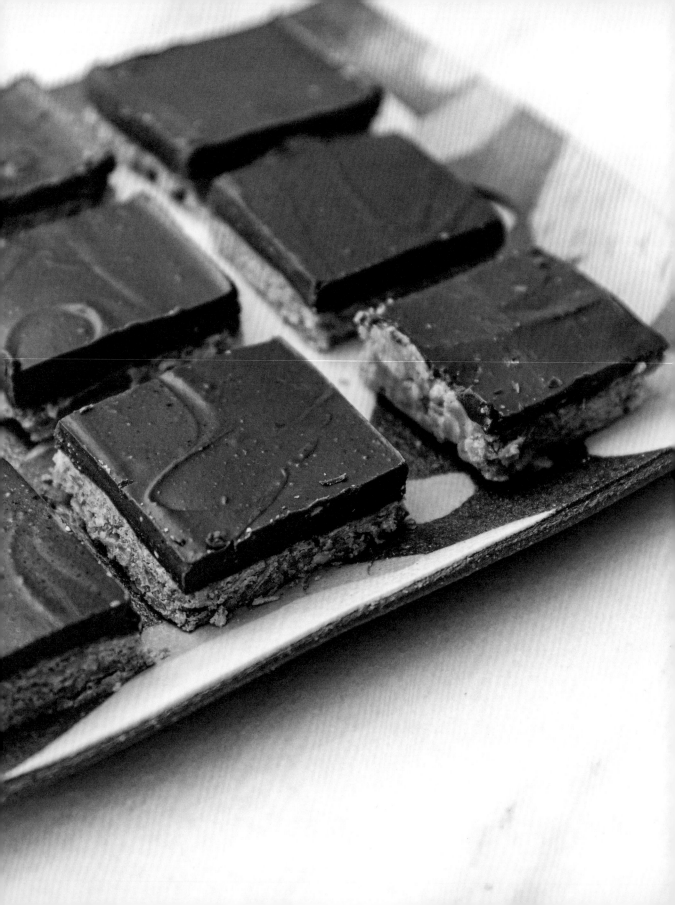

peanut butter bars

These super easy no-bake bars are my most requested item. They're amazingly simple to make but offer a complex set of flavors and very polished look, which doesn't happen nearly enough in life.

— MAKES 12 BARS —

FOR THE BARS:
2 cups (520 g) peanut butter
½ cup (120 ml) maple syrup
3 cups (270 g) gluten-free rolled oats

FOR THE CHOCOLATE GANACHE:
1½ cups (270 g) chocolate chips
3 tablespoons peanut butter
180 milligrams CBD oil

Line an 8 x 12-inch (20 x 30-cm) rectangular baking pan with parchment paper.

Make the bars: In a medium saucepan over low heat, combine the peanut butter and maple syrup and stir until smooth. Stir in the oats until thoroughly combined. Press the mixture firmly into the parchment-lined pan, making sure it's evenly distributed.

Make the ganache: In a small saucepan over low heat, melt the chocolate and peanut butter, stirring until smooth.

Dump the ganache evenly over the oat mixture, smoothing it out with a rubber spatula. While the chocolate is still wet, add CBD evenly and smooth again with spatula. Refrigerate for 4 to 6 hours before cutting.

GF
V

peanut butter brown rice squares

In college, I was charged with making Rice Krispies treats for some event. I didn't grow up making them or even eating them, and as I read the instructions I'd printed out (we still did that then), I was amazed at how butter and marshmallows became twice as delicious when melted together. Brown rice syrup and peanut butter are an equally delectable pairing in this more healthful take on a classic.

——————————— MAKES 12 SQUARES ———————————

¼ cup (65 g) peanut butter

4 ounces (120 ml) brown rice syrup

2 tablespoons maple syrup

1 tablespoon ground flaxseed

4 cups (105 g) gluten-free crispy brown rice cereal

1 cup (180 g) chocolate chips

180 milligrams CBD oil

Line an 8 x 12-inch (20 x 30-cm) baking pan with parchment paper.

In a medium-size saucepan over medium-low heat, heat the peanut butter and brown rice syrup until smooth and creamy. Remove from the heat, then add the maple syrup and ground flaxseed. Stir again before adding the rice cereal. Combine thoroughly and then add the chocolate chips.

Turn the mixture out into the baking pan, using clean hands to mold it into shape. Using a knife, gently score the lines of the squares before dosing each with 15 milligrams CBD oil. Cover and allow to set in the fridge for 2 to 4 hours or overnight.

GF

V

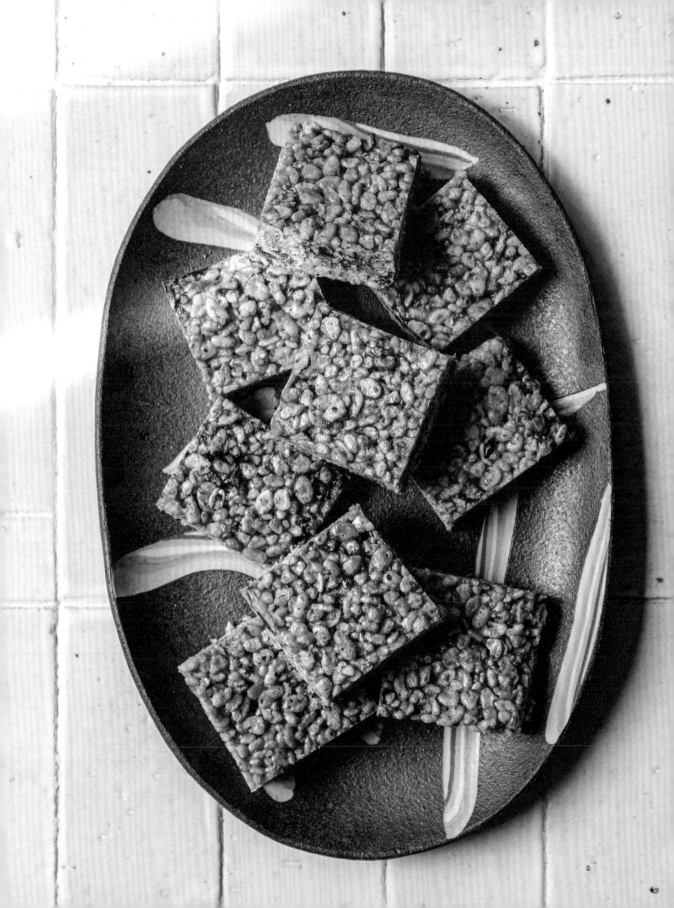

cookies, bars & cakes

rustic chocolate chip cookies

People love a good chocolate chip cookie. As a result, I have an arsenal of recipes. This is one of my favorites.

─────── **MAKES 24 COOKIES** ───────

⅔ cup (115 g) cultured vegan butter (page 28), melted

½ cup (65 g) coconut sugar

1 teaspoon pure vanilla extract

¼ teaspoon sea salt

2⅓ cups (170 g) almond flour

1 teaspoon baking soda

1 teaspoon baking powder

¼ cup (60 ml) maple syrup

1 cup (180 g) chocolate chips

360 milligrams CBD oil

Preheat the oven to 350° F (180° C) and line 2 baking sheets with parchment paper.

In a small saucepan over low heat, melt the cultured vegan butter. Transfer the melted butter to the bowl of a stand mixer or large, heavy-bottomed bowl. Add the coconut sugar and mix, then incorporate the vanilla and salt. Next, add the almond flour, baking soda and powder, mixing together for about 1 minute. Add the maple syrup, dampening the dough before folding in the chocolate chips.

Using a cookie scoop, scoop the dough to form 24 cookies and transfer to the parchment-lined baking sheets. Bake until browned at the edges, 10 to 12 minutes. Once you've removed the cookies from the oven, dose each with 4 drops (15 milligrams) of CBD oil (the warm cookies will absorb the oil).

GF

V

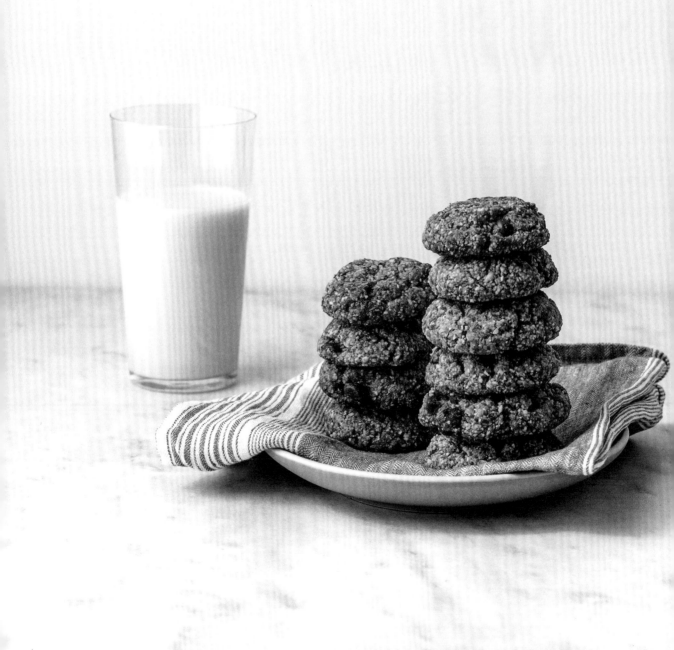

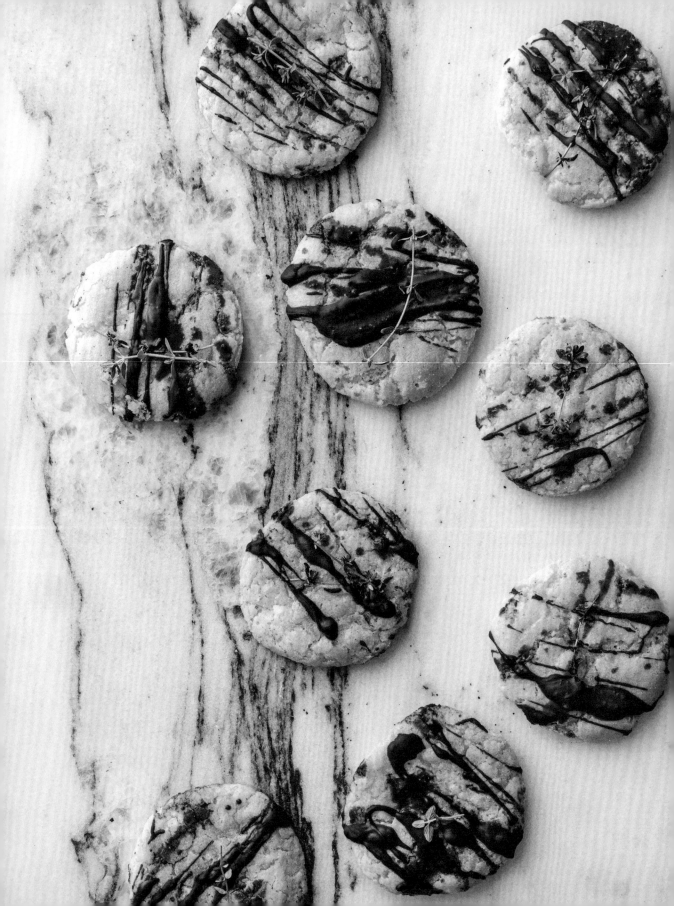

almond cookies

I use these cookies as pressed flower cookies and they're much prettier if they're very pale—which is why they're one of the few recipes that call for granulated sugar. If you don't have it, coconut sugar works fine, but the cookies will not be white. If you want to avoid gluten, make sure you purchase a gluten-free variety of almond paste. You can also make your own almond paste or buy it premade.

─────── **MAKES 11 COOKIES** ───────

7 ounces (200 g) almond paste

1 egg white

¼ teaspoon pure vanilla extract

⅔ cup (130 g) granulated sugar, plus more for serving (optional)

165 milligrams CBD oil

Hot fudge (page 168) and fresh thyme, for serving (optional)

Preheat the oven to 350° F (180° C) and line 2 baking sheets with parchment paper.

In the bowl of a stand mixer, beat the almond paste on high for a minute or two before adding the egg white, vanilla, and sugar. Beat on high for another minute. For each cookie, use a tablespoon to spoon dough into your clean hands and roll it into a ball. This is a very sticky dough so rinsing your hands with water before handling the dough will help keep them from sticking to your skin. Transfer to the parchment-lined baking sheets, spacing the cookies a bit to allow them to spread. Repeat to make 11 cookies.

Bake for 10 to 12 minutes, checking for golden coloring on the edges. After you remove the cookies from the oven (and before adding any toppings), dose each with 15 milligrams CBD oil.

Optionally, you can drizzle with hot fudge and garnish with fresh thyme.

GF

flat and chewy chocolate chip cookies

I have multiple chocolate chip cookie recipes because I really like chocolate chip cookies. As the name suggests, these bake up chewy and flat—my husband's favorite—and we usually have at least one batch around the house at all times. It helps that they freeze well.

MAKES 17 COOKIES

2 cups (180 g) blanched almond flour

¾ cup (30 g) almond flour

¼ cup (35 g) coconut sugar

½ teaspoon baking soda

½ teaspoon baking powder

¼ teaspoon sea salt

¼ cup (45 g) coconut oil, melted

½ cup (120 ml) maple syrup

1 teaspoon pure vanilla extract

½ cup (90 g) chocolate chips

255 milligrams CBD oil

Preheat the oven to 350° F (180° C) and line 2 baking sheets with parchment paper.

In the bowl of a stand mixer, use a fork to loosely combine the almond flours, coconut sugar, baking soda and powder, and salt. In a separate bowl, stir together the melted coconut oil, maple syrup, and vanilla; add dry ingredients to the wet ingredients a few tablespoons at a time to fully incorporate.

Using a 1-inch cookie scoop or a tablespoon, scoop the dough onto the parchment-lined sheets, leaving plenty of room between the cookies (they'll spread a bit). Bake cookies until lightly browned, checking to make sure they don't burn, 12 to 14 minutes. Remove from the oven and dose each cookie with 15 milligrams CBD oil (the warm cookies will absorb the oil). Allow the cookies to cool completely before removing them from the baking sheet, otherwise they'll break.

GF

V

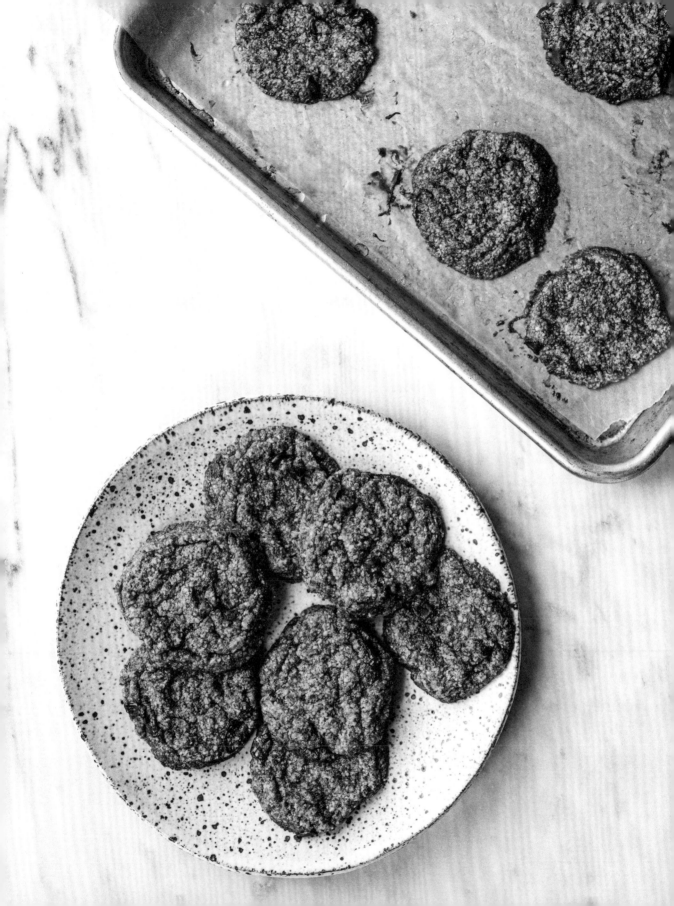

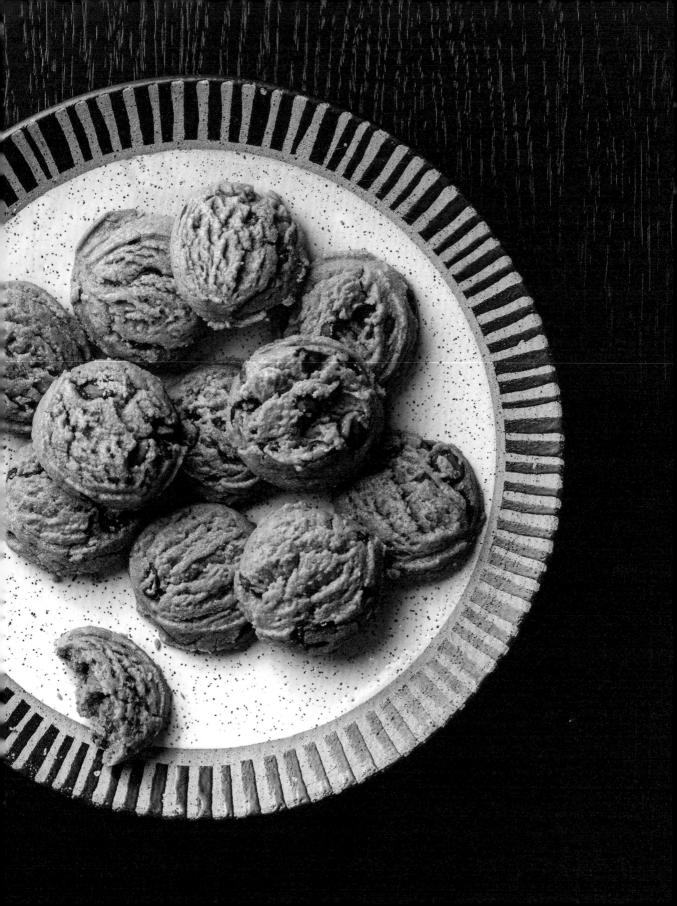

peanut butter cookies

I've been making this recipe for so long I'm not really sure where it came from at this point, but because these cookies are made with ingredients that are usually on hand, they're always easy to whip up. They're hearty and delicious and everyone loves them—even people who say they don't like peanut butter, which is just crazy.

—— MAKES 16 COOKIES ——

1 cup (260 g) peanut butter

¾ cup (105 g) coconut sugar

1 egg

½ teaspoon baking soda

¼ teaspoon sea salt

½ cup (90 g) chocolate chips

240 milligrams CBD oil

Preheat the oven to 350° F (180° C) and line 2 baking sheets with parchment paper.

In the bowl of a stand mixer, combine the peanut butter, coconut sugar, and egg. Beat on high for 2 minutes, then add the baking soda and salt. Churn for a minute or two more before folding in the chocolate chips.

Using a cookie scoop or tablespoon, scoop the dough onto the parchment-lined baking sheets. Bake until the cookies begin to darken a bit at the edges and around the chocolate chips, about 12 to 14 minutes.

Remove from the oven and dose each cookie with 15 milligrams CBD oil. Allow the cookies to cool completely before removing from the baking sheet.

GF

crispy oat thins

These are a healthier take on the classic slice-and-bake cookies my mother and grandmother make. But I'm too impatient to deal with the chilling and slicing, and my version uses heartier flours and fats as well as an unrefined sugar.

——————————————— MAKES ABOUT 24 COOKIES ———————————————

⅔ cup (115 g) cultured vegan butter (page 28)

2½ tablespoons coconut butter (page 25)

½ cup (65 g) coconut sugar

2 eggs

¼ cup (60 ml) maple syrup

1 teaspoon pure vanilla extract

1½ cups (135 g) gluten-free rolled oats

1 cup (90 g) blanched almond flour

¼ teaspoon fine sea salt

1 teaspoon baking powder

1 teaspoon baking soda

⅓ cup (50 g) raisins

⅓ cup (35 g) raw walnuts

4 ounces (95 g) dark vegan chocolate, coarsely chopped

360 milligrams CBD oil

Preheat the oven to 350° F (180° C) and line 2 baking sheets with parchment paper.

In a saucepan over low heat, melt both the butters (cultured vegan and coconut), stirring constantly. Transfer the melted butter to the bowl of a stand mixer, then beat in the coconut sugar, eggs, and maple syrup, followed by the vanilla.

In a separate bowl, whisk together the oats, almond flour, salt, baking powder and soda, and whisk before adding the dry ingredients to the wet and mixing together on low to medium for 1 to 2 minutes. Scrape down the bowl using a spatula and add the raisins, walnuts, and chocolate. Beat on medium to high for 1 minute—which is also a lazy (but effective) way to get bite-size bits of walnuts and chocolate without chopping.

Using a cookie scoop or tablespoon, scoop the dough onto the parchment-lined sheets, leaving at least a thumb-size space between each cookie. Bake until cookies turn golden around the edges, 12 to 13 minutes.

Remove from the oven, then dose each cookie with 15 milligrams CBD oil. Allow cookies to cool on sheets.

GF

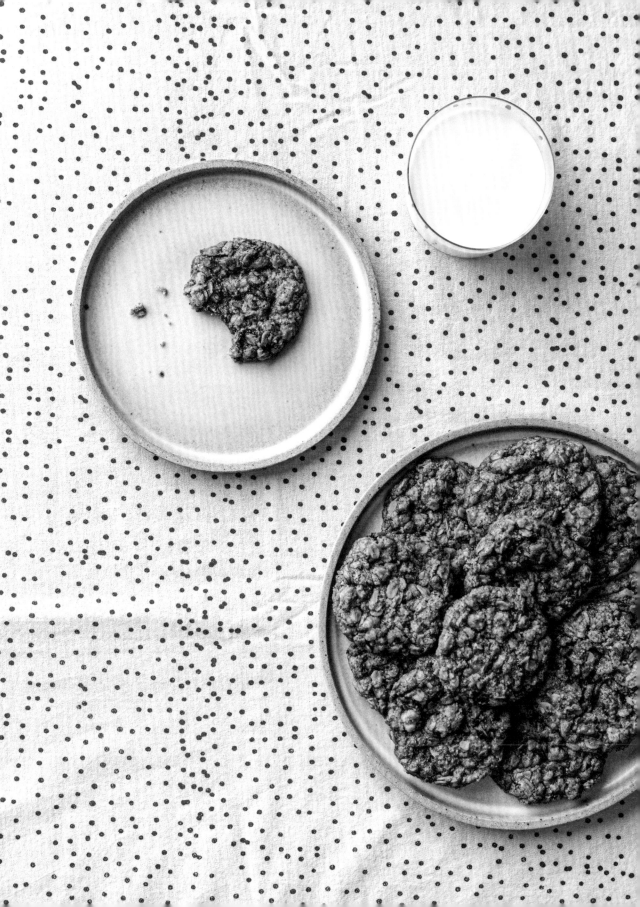

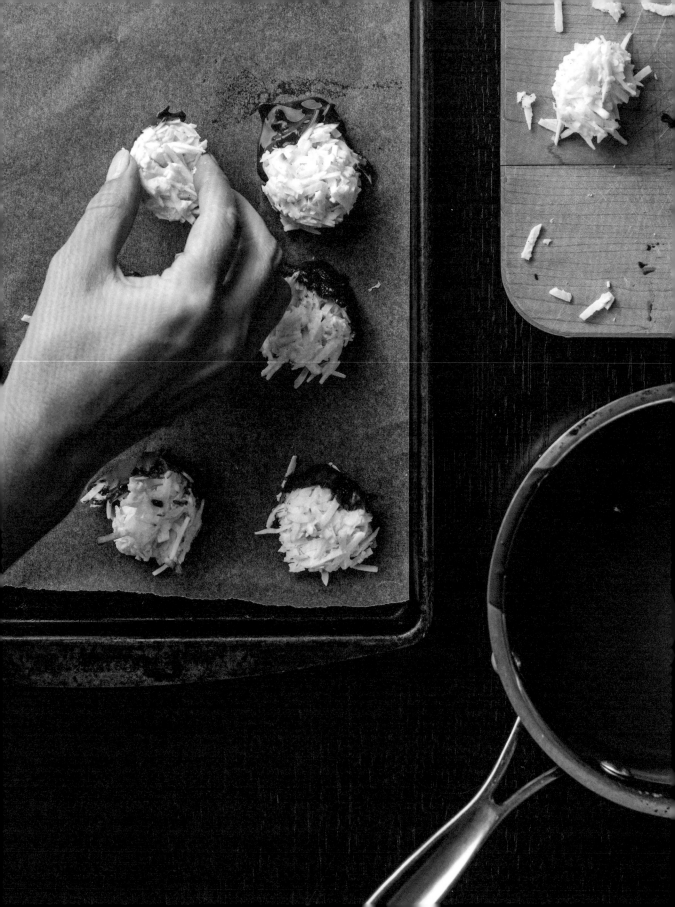

ketogenic lemon macaroons

Occasionally it's nice to have an alternative recipe on hand for people who don't do sugars—even unrefined sugars. I have more than a few of those friends and they're always thrilled when I bring something they, too, can eat.

— MAKES 18 MACAROONS —

5 egg whites

2½ cups (140 g) dessicated coconut

2 tablespoons coconut flour

1 teaspoon pure vanilla extract

3 sweet limes or Meyer lemons, zested and juiced

1 teaspoon almond extract

½ teaspoon stevia

¼ teaspoon sea salt

270 milligrams CBD oil

2 ounces (55 g) unsweetened dark chocolate (optional)

½ tablespoon coconut oil (optional)

Preheat the oven to 350° F (180° C). Line 2 baking sheets with parchment paper.

In the bowl of a stand mixer, beat the egg whites until stiff peaks form before adding the coconut and flour as well as the vanilla, lemon zest, and juice (I use a zester and then give both halves a good squeeze), almond extract, stevia, and salt. For each macaroon, spoon out a scant teaspoon of the foamy dough, trying to keep it as compact as possible on the parchment-lined sheets. Bake until the coconut gets a brownish glow at the edges, 10 to 12 minutes.

Remove from the oven and dose each macaroon with 15 milligrams CBD oil. Optionally, melt the dark chocolate and coconut oil in a small saucepan over low heat until fully incorporated and smooth. Dip half of each cookie immediately and allow them to fully cool before handling.

GF

cocoa pavlovas

The first time I made a successful soufflé it felt like a victory for latchkey kids worldwide with moms who didn't cook. I remember reading about a schoolteacher who said that kids were refreshing because they didn't know things were supposed to be scary or difficult. When you don't know that pastries might fail, it's just any other recipe, isn't it? These individual pavlovas—a mini version of the classic baked meringue dessert—look dainty and tricky but are deceptively easy.

MAKES 12 PAVLOVAS

4 egg whites

½ cup (35 g) cocoa powder

1 teaspoon pure vanilla extract

¼ teaspoon sea salt

3 cups (275 g) confectioner's sugar

1¾ cups (280 g) chocolate chips

180 milligrams CBD oil

Fresh berries, such as strawberries or blueberries, and whipped coconut cream, for serving (optional)

Preheat the oven to 350° F (180° C) and line a baking sheet with parchment paper.

In the bowl of a stand mixer (or using a hand mixer), beat the egg whites until foamy peaks form (about 2 to 3 minutes). Add cocoa powder 1 tablespoon at a time, beating gently. Beat in the vanilla and salt, followed by the confectioner's sugar, 1 cup at a time. Fold in the chocolate chips and the CBD oil, stirring with a spatula to incorporate evenly.

Using a cookie scoop or tablespoon, heap generous-size puffs of the mixture on the parchment paper (about 1½ tablespoons per cookie). Bake until golden brown and fluffy, 9 to 12 minutes. (They should look like large cream puffs; if they start to sink, stick them back in the oven for another minute or two.) Allow to cool completely, about 30 minutes. If you'd like, top with fresh berries and whipped coconut cream.

GF

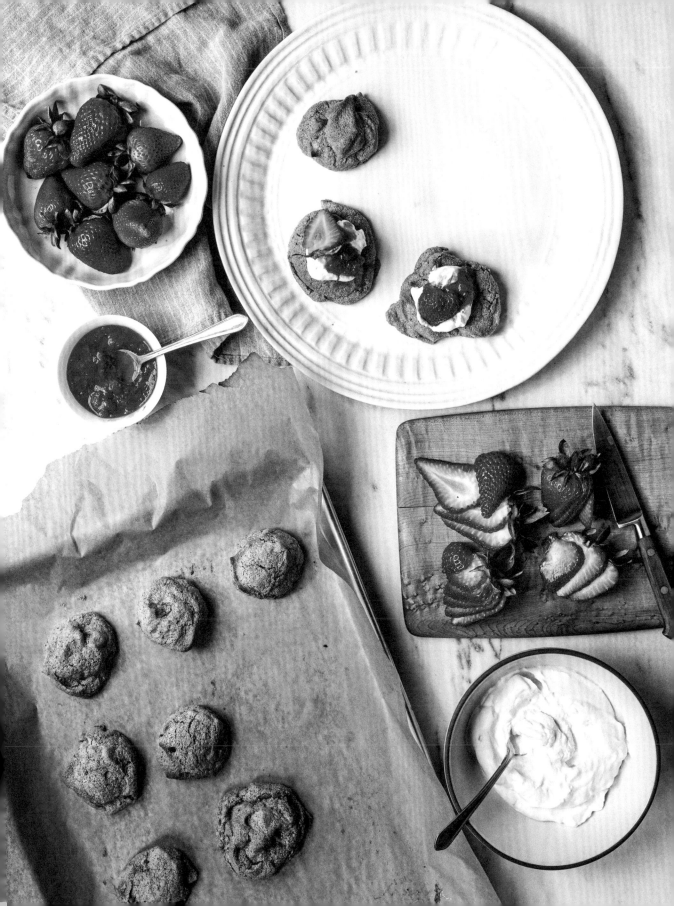

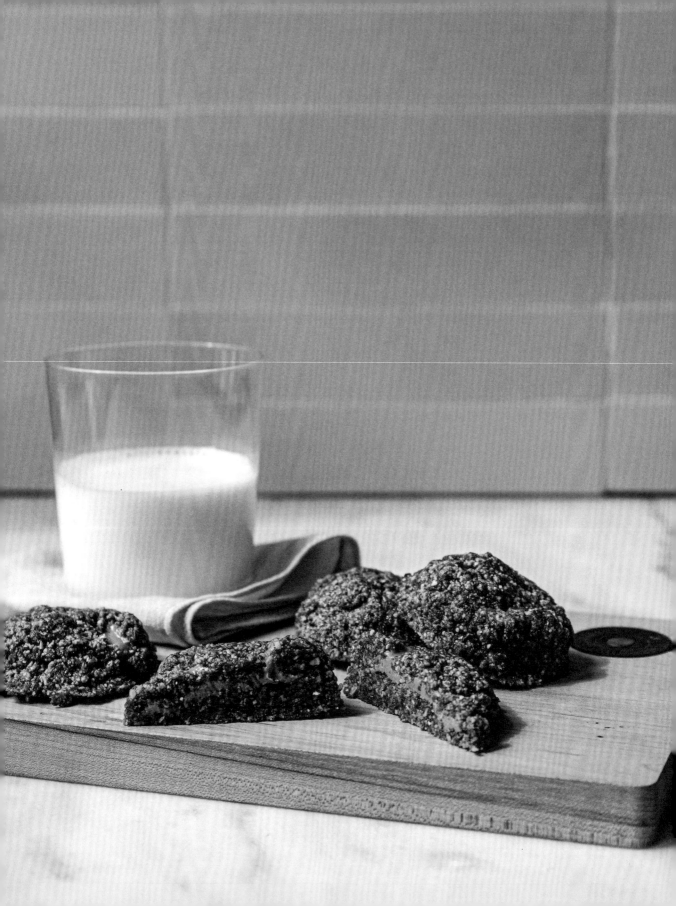

peanut butter bombs

This is hands down my favorite cookie. It's essentially a chocolate sugar cookie wrapped around a peanut butter center. Soft and satisfying. Everyone needs a warm peanut butter center sometimes.

———— **MAKES 9 TO 10 COOKIES** ————

FOR THE COOKIES:

⅓ cup (60 g) cultured vegan butter (page 28)

⅓ cup (60 g) coconut butter (page 25)

½ cup (65 g) coconut sugar

1 egg

2 teaspoons cocoa powder

1 teaspoon pure vanilla extract

1 teaspoon salt

2 cups (165 g) almond meal

¼ cup (60 ml) maple syrup

FOR THE PEANUT BUTTER FILLING:

¾ cup (195 g) peanut butter

2 tablespoons maple syrup

150 milligrams CBD oil

Preheat the oven to 350° F (180° C) and line a baking sheet with parchment paper.

Make the cookies: In the bowl of a stand mixer, combine the vegan butter, coconut butter, and coconut sugar and mix on medium for 1 minute. Add the egg and mix again for 1 minute before adding the cocoa powder, vanilla, and salt. Mix again for 1 minute, then mix in the almond meal and maple syrup.

Make the peanut butter filling: In a separate bowl, mix the peanut butter, maple syrup, and CBD and stir until fully combined.

For each cookie, use a cookie scoop or a tablespoon to measure a ball of dough and place on clean, damp hands. Flatten the chocolate dough like a pancake in one hand, and using the other, scoop a very scant tablespoon of peanut butter filling into the center, like a dumpling. Gently close the chocolate cookie around the peanut butter and place on the parchment-lined sheet. Repeat to make 9 to 10 cookies.

Bake for 10 to 12 minutes, until cookies look slightly firm and slightly lighter on the edges.

GF

spirulina mint chip "grasshopper" bars

Served cold, these bars are a summer favorite. They are a great way to use the mint we grow in spades around our home in Los Angeles, and also include spirulina, a powerful antioxidant, and peppermint oil, which is calming on the stomach and psyche.

— SERVES 6 —

FOR THE CRUST:
¾ cup (115 g) raw cashews
2 tablespoons cocoa powder
2 tablespoons coconut butter (page 25)
1 tablespoon maple syrup

FOR THE FILLING:
1½ cups (225 g) raw cashews
¼ cup (60 ml) maple syrup
¼ cup (60 ml) coconut cream
3 tablespoons coconut oil

⅛ teaspoon peppermint extract
Handful of mint leaves (optional)
2 tablespoons cocoa nibs
¼ teaspoon sea salt
¼ teaspoon spirulina powder
1 teaspoon pure vanilla extract
90 milligrams CBD oil
2 ounces (55 g) unsweetened dark chocolate (optional)
½ tablespoon coconut oil (optional)

Line a 5 x 7-inch (13 x 18-cm) mini rectangular baking pan with parchment paper.

Make the crust: In a food processor, combine the cashews, cocoa powder, coconut butter, and maple syrup and process for 2 minutes. Using clean hands, press the dough into the parchment-lined pan.

Make the filling: In a high-speed blender, combine the cashews, maple syrup, coconut cream, coconut oil, peppermint extract, mint leaves (if using them) cocoa nibs, sea salt, spirulina powder, vanilla, and CBD oil and process on high until smooth and green, 2 to 3 minutes.

Turn the filling out into the pan, layered over the chocolate crust, and freeze for 4 to 6 hours. Optionally, melt the dark chocolate and ½ tablespoon coconut oil in a small saucepan over low heat and stir until fully incorporated and smooth. Drizzle over the frozen bars for a more polished look.

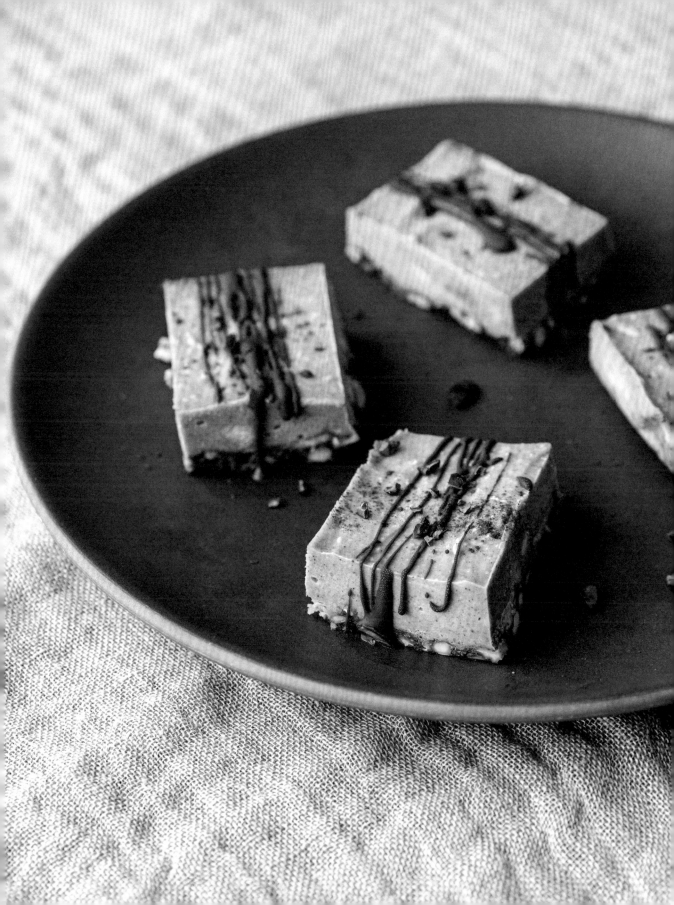

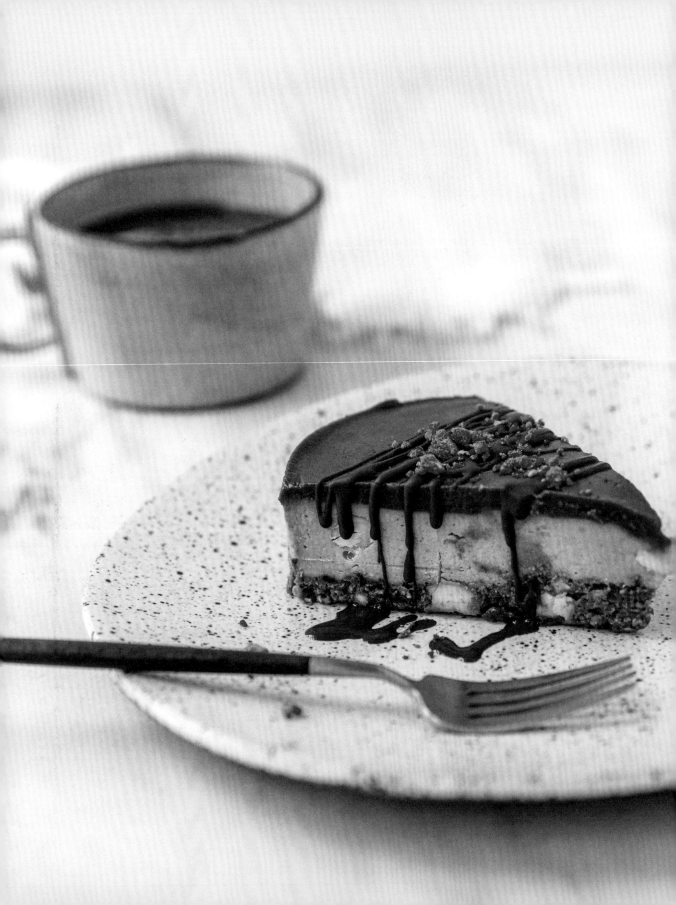

sweet beet treat

For a few years now I've been slightly obsessed with the color of beets. As far as I'm concerned, the fact that beets have antioxidant properties and support brain and digestive health is just a bonus, because they make everything terrifically beautiful with their natural bright magenta coloring.

— SERVES 6 —

FOR THE CRUST:
½ cup (75 g) raw cashews
½ cup (45 g) gluten-free rolled oats
4 dates, pitted
2 tablespoons cocoa powder
1 tablespoon maple syrup
1½ tablespoons coconut oil
¼ teaspoon pure vanilla extract

**FOR THE FIRST LAYER
OF FILLING:**
1 cup (150 g) raw cashews
½ cup (120 ml) maple syrup
¼ cup (60 ml) beet juice*

¼ cup (60 ml) coconut cream
1 lemon, juiced and zested
1 teaspoon pure vanilla extract
¼ teaspoon almond extract
¼ teaspoon sea salt

**FOR THE SECOND LAYER
OF FILLING:**
¼ cup (60 ml) maple syrup
2 tablespoons coconut butter
(page 25), melted
1 tablespoon cocoa powder
½ teaspoon pure vanilla extract
90 milligrams CBD oil

Line a 6-inch (15-cm) springform pan with parchment paper and grease with coconut oil.

Make the crust: In a food processor, process all the crust ingredients (cashews, oats, dates, cocoa powder, maple syrup, coconut oil, and vanilla extract) and blend until a coarse, sticky meal forms, about 2 minutes. Press the crust into the prepared pan and shape, molding crust with your hands to fill the bottom fully.

Make the filling: In a high-speed blender, combine all the ingredients for the first layer (cashews, maple syrup, beet juice, coconut cream, lemon, vanilla, almond, and salt) and blend on medium speed for 2 minutes. Pour mixture over the crust and scrape down the sides of the blender before moving on to the second layer. In the same blender, combine all ingredients, except the CBD oil, for the second layer (maple syrup, melted coconut butter, cocoa powder, and vanilla) and blend on high for 2 minutes or so.

Scrape the second layer of filling onto the top of the others in the pan and add the CBD oil, smoothing and distributing evenly with the back of a spoon. Refrigerate for at least 4 hours, removing the cake 15 minutes before cutting and serving it.

You can also toss a thumbnail-size chunk of peeled, raw beet directly into the blender.

(GF)
(V)

special cbd brownies

These no-bake brownies can be made in minutes in a blender or food processor and just a short stay in the freezer to set. They rely on tasty (and beneficial) spices and flavors, including cocoa powder, which is rich in polyphenols and improves blood flow to the brain, and cinnamon, which lowers blood sugar levels—as well as CBD.

MAKES 12 BROWNIES

FOR THE FIRST LAYER:

1 cup (90 g) gluten-free rolled oats

¾ cup (75 g) raw walnuts

4 dates, pitted

3 tablespoons melted coconut butter (page 25)

3 tablespoons cocoa powder

2 tablespoons ground flaxseed

1 teaspoon pure vanilla extract

½ teaspoon ground cinnamon

¼ teaspoon sea salt

½ cup (120 ml) coconut cream

FOR THE FROSTING:

3 tablespoons maple syrup

2 tablespoons cocoa powder

1 tablespoon coconut butter (page 25)

2 tablespoons peanut butter (or almond butter)

180 milligrams CBD oil

Line a 5 x 7-inch (13 x 18-cm) mini rectangular baking pan with parchment paper.

Make the first layer: In a food processor or high-speed blender, combine the rolled oats, walnuts, dates, melted coconut butter, cocoa powder, flaxseed, vanilla, cinnamon, and sea salt (everything but the coconut cream), and blend quickly, about 50 seconds to 1 minute, moving from low to high (if using a blender). Next, add the coconut cream and blend.

Pour the mixture into the parchment-lined pan and, using clean hands, press the dough into the pan, smoothing it out to be evenly distributed.

Make the frosting: Rinse out the blender. Combine the maple syrup, cocoa powder, coconut butter, and nut butter and blend on high for 2 minutes before scraping out into a bowl. Add the CBD and stir evenly before frosting the brownies with a rubber spatula. Freeze for at least 2 hours, then gently run a butter knife along the sides of the pan to remove before cutting.

GF

V

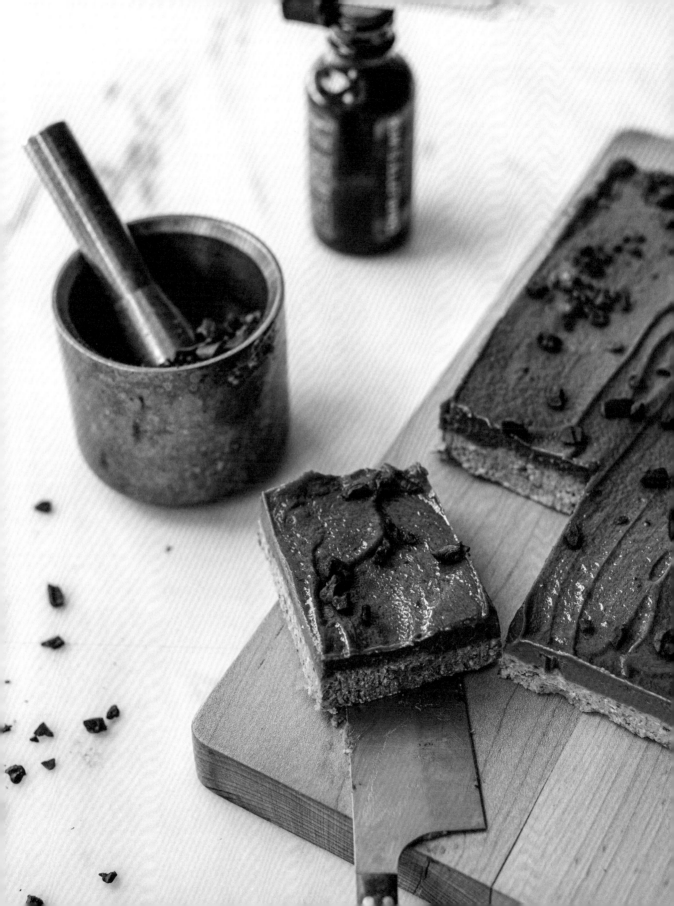

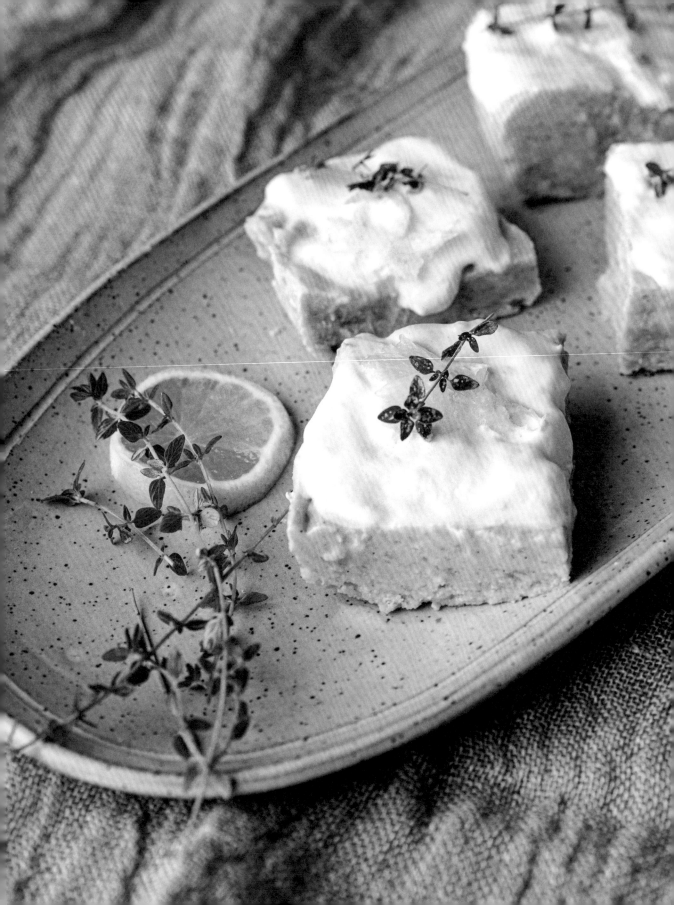

lemon bars with coconut crust

These were always a staple of my childhood—lemon bars with a shortbread situation. This version is more like an icebox cake, and instead of shortbread it has a coconut base, which complements the lemon flavor and works well for nondairy eaters avoiding butter. The recipe also calls for agar-agar—a vegetarian alternative to gelatin. The bars can be topped with aquafaba whipped cream (brine retained from a can of chickpeas whipped with vanilla and a dash of powdered sugar), or real whipped cream (if you eat it) for a pretty finish.

_____ MAKES 6 BARS _____

FOR THE CRUST:

3 tablespoons coconut flour

¼ cup (25 g) gluten-free rolled oats

3½ tablespoons coconut butter (page 25)

¼ cup (60 ml) maple syrup

¼ teaspoon sea salt

FOR THE FILLING:

2 lemons, zested and juiced

2 teaspoons agar-agar flakes

½ cup (110 g) vegan yogurt (page 26)

¼ cup (60 ml) maple syrup

3 tablespoons coconut cream

1 teaspoon pure vanilla extract

90 milligrams CBD oil

Aquafaba whipped cream or dairy whipped cream, for serving (optional)

Preheat the oven to 350° F (180° C) and line a 5 x 7-inch (13 x 18-cm) mini rectangular baking pan with parchment paper and grease with coconut oil.

Make the crust: In a food processor, blend the coconut flour, oats, coconut butter, maple syrup, and salt until a coarse meal forms. Using clean hands, press it into the parchment-lined pan and up the sides.

Bake until the crust is golden brown, 12 to 15 minutes.

Meanwhile, make the filling: In a small saucepan over low heat, stir together the lemon zest and juice, agar-agar, yogurt, maple syrup, coconut cream, and vanilla. Remove from the heat and add the CBD oil. Allow the mixture to cool to room temperature before pouring the filling into the prepared crust. Freeze for 4 to 6 hours. Use a sharp knife to cut into 6 squares, top with whipped cream if using, and serve immediately.

GF

V

brownies à la hoy

For a few months I made vegan, gluten-free meals for some friends and fellow moms (many of whom are *both* friends and fellow moms). These brownies were created for a wonderful working mama with a sweet tooth and a lot of the input was all hers. She wanted a lower sugar/carb situation, and the result was dense and delicious—almost like a flourless chocolate pavé.

———————————— MAKES 6 BROWNIES ————————————

3 ounces (70 g) unsweetened dark chocolate

¼ cup (60 ml) coconut cream

½ cup (120 ml) maple syrup

¼ cup (65 g) peanut butter

1½ teaspoons pure vanilla extract

1 cup (80 g) almond flour

2 tablespoons (15 g) coconut flour

2 teaspoons baking powder

90 milligrams CBD oil

Preheat the oven to 350° F (180° C) and line a 5 x 7-inch (13 x 18-cm) baking pan with parchment paper.

In a small saucepan over low heat, gently heat the chocolate, adding the maple syrup and coconut cream, followed by the peanut butter and vanilla, stirring until smooth. Remove from the heat, then stir in both the flours and baking powder before adding the CBD oil.

Spread the mixture evenly in the parchment-lined pan. Bake until brownies start to brown (keep an eye on them to make sure they don't burn), 35 to 40 minutes.

Let the brownies cool for at least 45 minutes before handling, allowing them to set.

GF

V

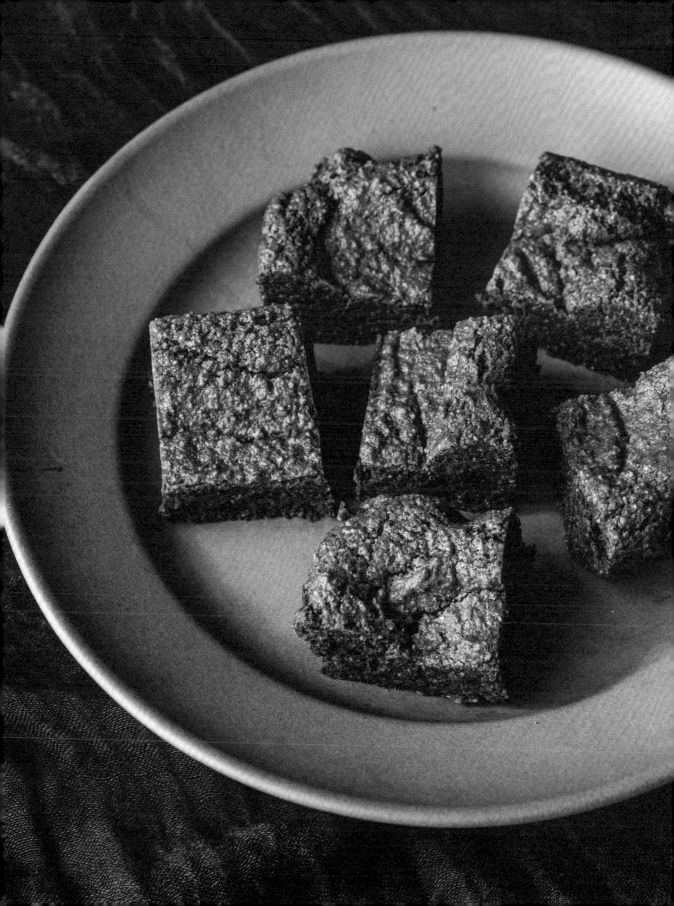

CAKES

carrot cake

When I was growing up, there was a tiny cafe in the next town over that served a towering, crumbling, deliciously messy carrot cake filled with walnuts and coconut and generously iced with cream cheese frosting. I'd beg my mother to take me for *the* carrot cake—this unique and artisanal version filled with recognizable components of the whole, which nobody else seemed to serve without the pedestrian orange carrot made with icing on top. Mine doesn't tower, but in every other way it's fairly spot-on. This cake also has fiber, fruits, and nuts to keep blood sugar levels in check and leave you feeling full and satisfied in all the right ways.

―――― **MAKES ONE 9 X 12-INCH (23 X 30-CM) CAKE (ABOUT 24 SMALL SERVINGS)** ――――

FOR THE CAKE:
1½ cups (185 g) shredded carrots

½ cup (50 g) shredded coconut flakes

½ cup (85 g) dried apricots

1 tablespoon raisins

⅓ cup (30 g) raw almonds

3½ cups (280 g) almond flour

3 teaspoons baking powder

1 teaspoon baking soda

1 teaspoon sea salt

3 teaspoons ground cinnamon

1 teaspoon ground nutmeg

1 cup (240 ml) coconut milk

1 cup (240 ml) maple syrup

½ cup (100 g) cultured vegan butter (page 28), melted

3 tablespoons ground flaxseed

360 milligrams CBD oil

Vanilla frosting (page 174) and toasted coconut, for serving (optional)

Preheat the oven to 350° F (180° C). Line a 9 x 12-inch (23 x 30-cm) rectangular cake pan with parchment paper and grease with coconut oil.

In a food processor, grate the carrots, then add the coconut flakes, dried apricots, raisins, and almonds. Process for several minutes until mixture is damp and all is loosely incorporated, then transfer to the bowl of a stand mixer. Add the almond flour, baking powder, baking soda, salt, cinnamon, nutmeg, coconut milk, maple syrup, and melted vegan butter; mix for about 2 minutes.

In a small bowl, combine flaxseed with 5 tablespoons of warm water. Allow to sit for 5 minutes, then add flax and any remaining water to stand mixer bowl; mix to incorporate.

Spread the mixture into the prepared pan and bake until a toothpick inserted in the center comes out clean, 40 to 45 minutes. Remove from the oven and immediately dose the warm

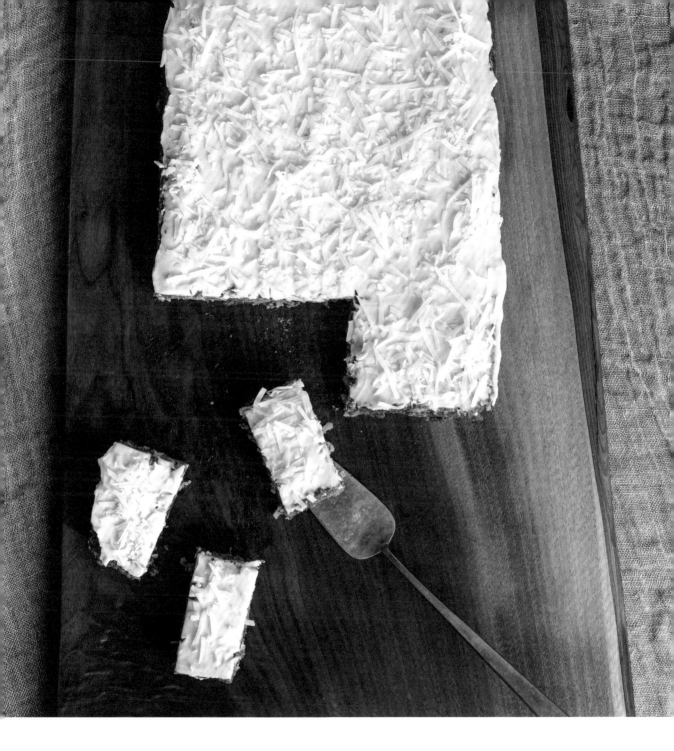

cake with the CBD oil. Allow the cake to cool on the counter, about 1 hour, then transfer to the refrigerator and chill for 2 to 3 hours or so (this will allow the CBD to be absorbed by the cake), before running a knife around the edges. When inverting it onto a cake board or large platter, cover the top of the pan with the plate and flip it, removing the parchment after.

Ice with vanilla frosting and sprinkle with toasted coconut.

almond, rosemary, and olive oil cake

This cake is simple and hearty. At my house we use it as a breakfast cake, heaping it with everything from berries to crumbled nuts and powdered sugar. It's very moist and moves through the seasons with astounding versatility.

MAKES ONE 9-INCH (23-CM) CAKE (ABOUT 9 SERVINGS)

3 cups (270 g) blanched almond flour

¼ teaspoon sea salt

1½ teaspoons baking soda

3 large eggs

2 tablespoons nut milk (page 20 or 23)

¼ cup (60 ml) maple syrup

2 tablespoons coconut sugar

½ cup (120 ml) cashew cream (page 27)

½ cup (120 ml) olive oil

2 lemons, zested and juiced

1 teaspoon chopped rosemary

135 milligrams CBD oil

Vanilla frosting (page 174), or lemon zest and confectioner's sugar, for serving (optional)

Preheat the oven to 350° F (180° C) and line a 9-inch (23-cm) springform baking pan with parchment paper measured and cut to fit the bottom. Grease the rest of the pan (including parchment) with olive oil.

In a large bowl, mix the flour, salt and baking soda. In the bowl of a stand mixer, combine the eggs, nut milk, maple syrup, coconut sugar, cashew cream, olive oil, lemon zest and juice, rosemary, and CBD oil. Mix thoroughly on high for 2 minutes before slowly incorporating the dry ingredients.

Transfer the cake batter to the oiled pan and bake until a toothpick inserted in the center comes out clean, 35 to 40 minutes. Allow to cool for 45 minutes, then run a butter knife around the edges before releasing the cake from the springform pan. Cut into slices and enjoy.

Optionally, you can frost the cake with vanilla frosting or dust with confectioner's sugar and lemon zest if you want to dress it up a little, though plain is fine, too.

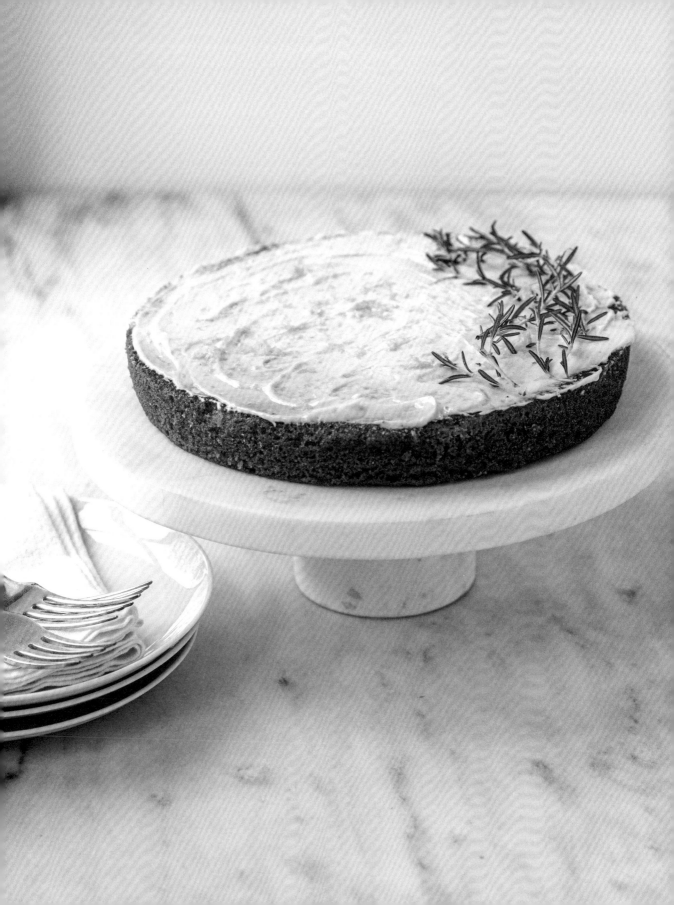

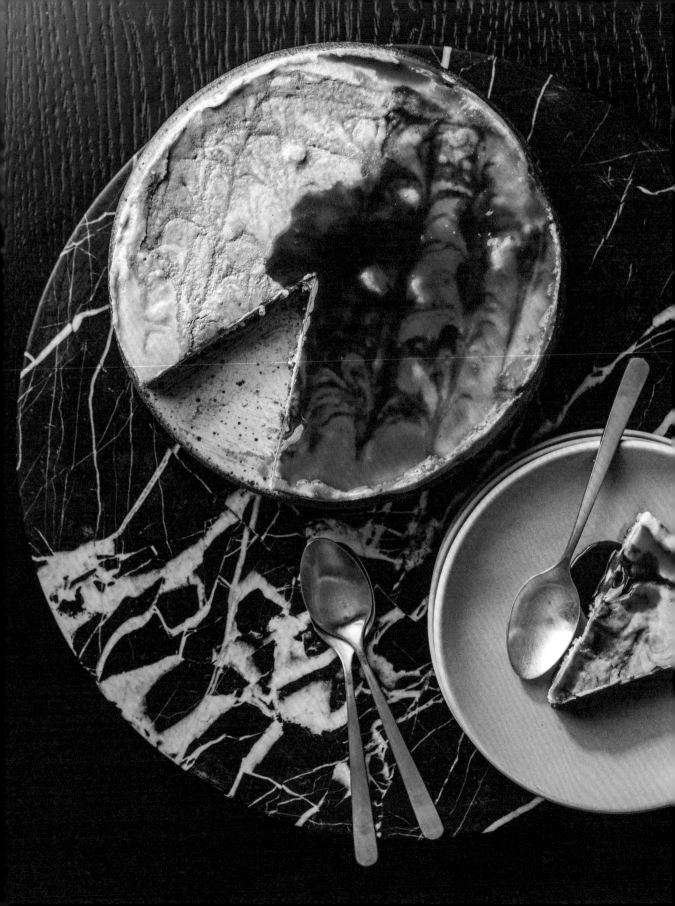

blue butterfly tea "cheesecake"

Blue butterfly pea flowers are said to improve eyesight, hair growth, and skin quality as well as being an antioxidant. They're also the most gorgeous color, so it makes sense to marble the tea into a cake that might also make you more beautiful.

MAKES ONE 9-INCH (23-CM) CAKE (ABOUT 9 SERVINGS)

FOR THE CRUST:

1 cup (90 g) gluten-free rolled oats

½ cup (50 g) raw walnuts

2 tablespoons maple syrup

1 tablespoon coconut butter (page 25)

5 dates, pitted

¼ teaspoon sea salt

FOR THE CAKE:

½ cup (120 ml) steeped blue butterfly chai tea

1 cup (240 ml) coconut cream

¼ cup (60 ml) maple syrup

1 teaspoon pure vanilla extract

1⅓ cups (180 g) raw cashews

135 milligrams CBD oil

Line a 9-inch (23-cm) springform baking pan with parchment paper measured and cut to fit the bottom, then grease the rest of the pan (including parchment) with coconut oil.

Make the crust: In a food processor, blend the oats, walnuts, maple syrup, coconut butter, pitted dates, and salt until a rough paste forms. Using clean, damp hands, mold the crust to the oiled pan.

Make the cake: In a high-speed blender, mix the steeped and slightly cooled tea with the coconut cream, maple syrup, and vanilla, and blend on high for 2 minutes; add the cashews and CBD oil, blending just until fully incorporated. Pour the filling into the prepared pan and spread evenly over the crust. Freeze for 4 to 6 hours before running a knife around the edges and releasing the springform pan. The cake can be pulled off the bottom of the pan and placed on a serving plate when frozen.

Allow the cake to sit at room temperature for 10 to 15 minutes before cutting.

(GF)
(V)

turmeric baked "cheesecake"

Early on in my baking orders I had someone request I make a cake version of a turmeric latte. This was the resulting recipe and I've never had any complaints. Like the latte, it's filled with spices and flavors to keep your insides in good function while satisfying any sweet tooth.

————————— **MAKES ONE TART (ABOUT 7 SERVINGS)** —————————

FOR THE CRUST:
1 cup (150 g) raw cashews
5 dates, pitted
1 tablespoon maple syrup
1 tablespoon coconut oil
1 teaspoon pure vanilla extract
¼ teaspoon sea salt

FOR THE CAKE:
1 cup (150 g) raw cashews
½ cup (110 g) cashew yogurt (page 26)

½ cup (120 ml) maple syrup
1 tablespoon ground flaxseed
1 teaspoon sea salt
1 teaspoon almond extract
1 teaspoon pure vanilla extract
¼ teaspoon ground turmeric
½ teaspoon ground cinnamon
¼ teaspoon ground cardamom
105 milligrams CBD oil

Preheat the oven to 350° F (180° C). Generously oil a large rectangular tart mold with a removable bottom.

Make the crust: In a food processor, combine all the crust ingredients (cashews, dates, maple syrup, coconut oil, vanilla, and salt) and pulse until a crumbly mixture forms. Press into the oiled tart pan, making sure to climb the sides a little with your crust materials. Bake for 12 minutes.

Make the cake: In a high-speed blender, mix together the cashews, yogurt, maple syrup, flaxseed, salt, almond extract, vanilla, turmeric, cinnamon, and cardamom, blending until smooth and evenly incorporated. Pour batter into the crust, using a spatula to scrape down the sides of the blender and smooth the mixture in the cake pan and dose with the CBD oil. Bake until both the crust and top of cake begin to darken to golden, 25 to 30 minutes, checking to make sure the top doesn't burn.

Allow to cool for at least a half an hour before pushing the bottom of the tart mold out and running a knife along the edges of the pan to release the tart from the mold, sliding it onto a plate or board to serve.

(GF)
(V)

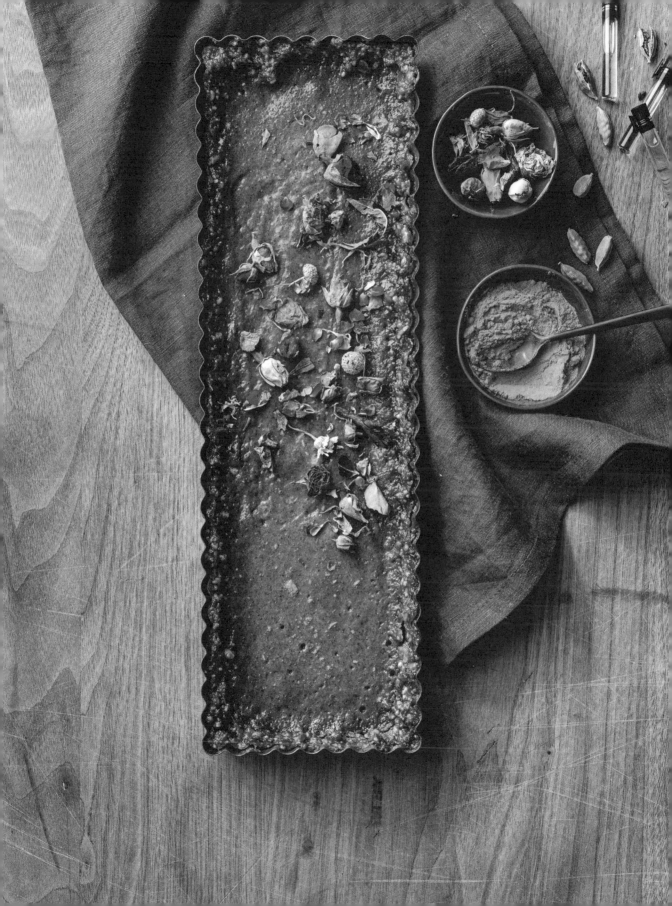

dense freezer cake

I was raised on ice cream cakes: dirt cake, Baskin-Robbins, and even this strange Dairy Queen frozen pizza dessert you could order from the drive-through. The best part about frozen cakes is how easy they are to make—especially when you're working with adaptogens and compounds you don't want to overheat. Wholesome additions like cocoa powder and almond butter also make it a rather guilt-free, but decadent, treat.

——————— MAKES ONE 9-INCH (23-CM) CAKE (ABOUT 9 SERVINGS) ———————

FOR THE CRUST:

2 cups (180 g) gluten-free rolled oats

12 dates, pitted

2 tablespoons coconut oil

½ teaspoon sea salt

1 teaspoon pure vanilla extract

FOR THE CAKE:

1 (13.5-ounce / 380-ml) can coconut milk

1 cup (150 g) raw cashews

½ cup (65 g) coconut sugar

½ cup (120 ml) maple syrup

3½ tablespoons almond butter

3 tablespoons cocoa powder

1 teaspoon almond extract

1 teaspoon pure vanilla extract

135 milligrams CBD oil

FOR THE TOPPING:

½ cup (90 g) chocolate chips

2 tablespoons almond butter

2 tablespoons coconut milk

Line a 9-inch (23-cm) springform pan with parchment paper (measured and cut to fit the bottom), and grease the sides generously with coconut oil.

Make the crust: In a food processor, combine all crust ingredients and blend until a paste forms. Using clean hands, press the crust into the parchment-lined pan.

Assemble the cake: In a high-speed blender or food processor, combine all cake ingredients, mixing on high until smooth, 2 to 3 minutes. Pour the mixture over the crust and jiggle it to ensure that it's even. Freeze for at least 4 hours before running a knife along the edges and releasing the springform to remove the cake. Set on a rack (keeping the metal springform bottom in place for easy moving).

Assemble the topping layer by melting the chocolate chips and almond butter on low heat in a small saucepan, stirring continuously. Add the coconut milk to thin the mixture a bit, then gently spoon over the top of the cake so it dribbles down the sides. Allow the cake to freeze again (a half hour or so), until the topping has set.

When you're ready to serve the cake, remove the bottom springform piece while the cake is still frozen and transfer to a cake plate. Serve within 30 to 40 minutes at most to ensure it doesn't get too melted.

GF

V

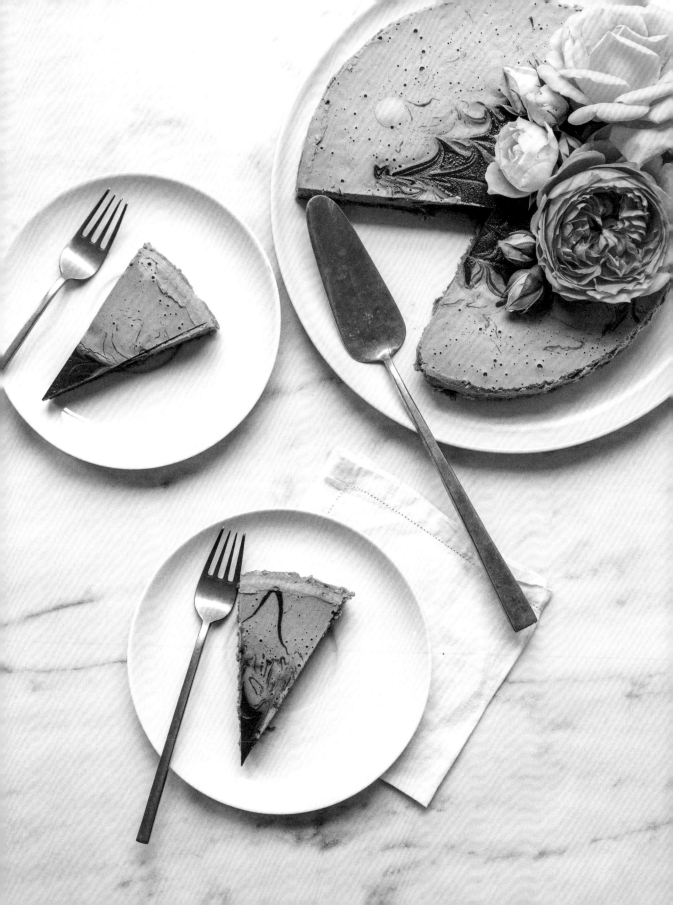

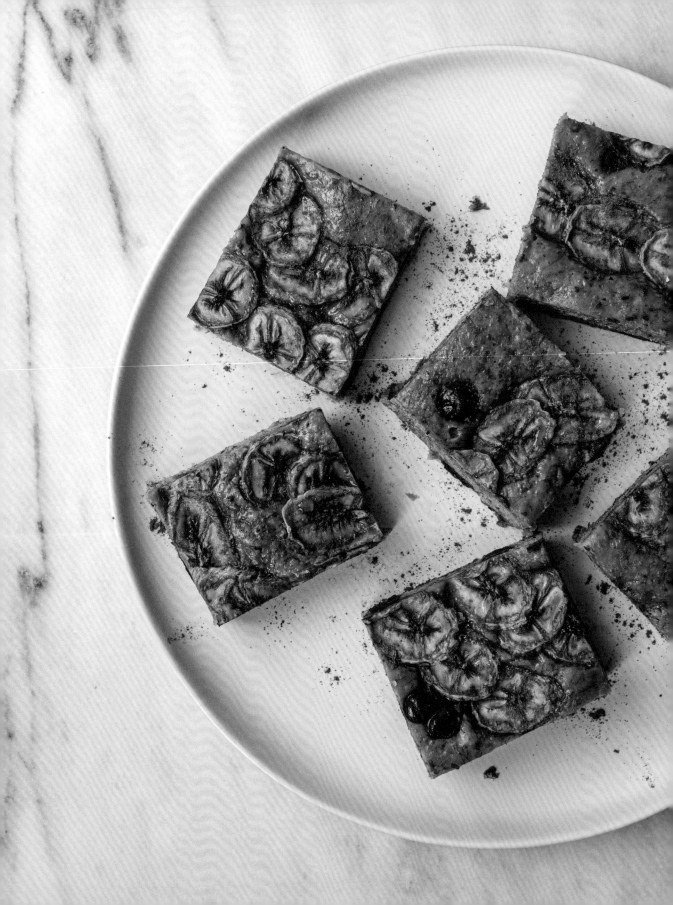

banana cake

This is a versatile cake that can be dressed either up or down, eaten for breakfast or saved for dessert. You can add chocolate chips or drench it in caramel sauce or leave it plain with some sliced bananas on top—either way, it's rich, moist, easy.

MAKES ONE 9-INCH (23-CM) CAKE (ABOUT 9 SERVINGS)

½ cup (65 g) coconut sugar

3 tablespoons maple syrup

3 ripe bananas

¼ cup (60 ml) coconut milk

2 lemons, juiced

¾ teaspoon baking soda

¼ teaspoon sea salt

1 cup (120 g) all-purpose flour

½ cup (40 g) almond flour

½ cup (90 g) chocolate chips (optional)

135 milligrams CBD oil

1 banana, sliced (optional)

Preheat the oven to 350° F (180° C) and grease a 9-inch (23-cm) springform pan with coconut oil.

In the bowl of a stand mixer, combine the coconut sugar, maple syrup, and the bananas, mixing on medium to high until incorporated. Add the coconut milk, lemon juice, baking soda, and salt, followed by the flours incrementally (about a half cup or so at a time); mix until fully incorporated, then add the CBD and stir. If you want to add chocolate chips, do so now, then scrape down the sides and mix again before turning out batter into the pan.

Optionally, you can arrange the sliced bananas on top or you can make a glaze using the caramel sauce recipe (page 168).

Bake until a toothpick inserted in the center comes out clean, 40 to 50 minutes.

pies & tarts

tarte au chocolat

This is a deceptively simple recipe. It usually fools anyone into thinking it's a traditional chocolate- and cream-filled dessert, when in fact it's dairy-free and works for most dietary restrictions. It's also filled with probiotic and healthy fat-centric coconut yogurt and cocoa powder to keep your brain fast moving.

———————— MAKES ONE 9-INCH (23-CM) TART (ABOUT 9 SERVINGS) ————————

1 (13.5-ounce / 380-ml) can coconut milk

1 cup (220 g) coconut yogurt

1 cup (130 g) coconut sugar

3 tablespoons cocoa powder

2 teaspoons agar-agar flakes

1 teaspoon pure vanilla extract

135 milligrams CBD oil

1 vegan piecrust (page 30)

Hot fudge (page 168), for serving (optional)

In a medium-size saucepan over low heat, combine the coconut milk, yogurt, sugar, cocoa powder, agar-agar, and vanilla. Heat, stirring, until the sugar dissolves and the ingredients combine. Remove from the heat and stir in the CBD oil. Pour into the prepared pie shell and refrigerate for at least 4 hours. If using, drizzle hot fudge for a more polished look before cutting into slices.

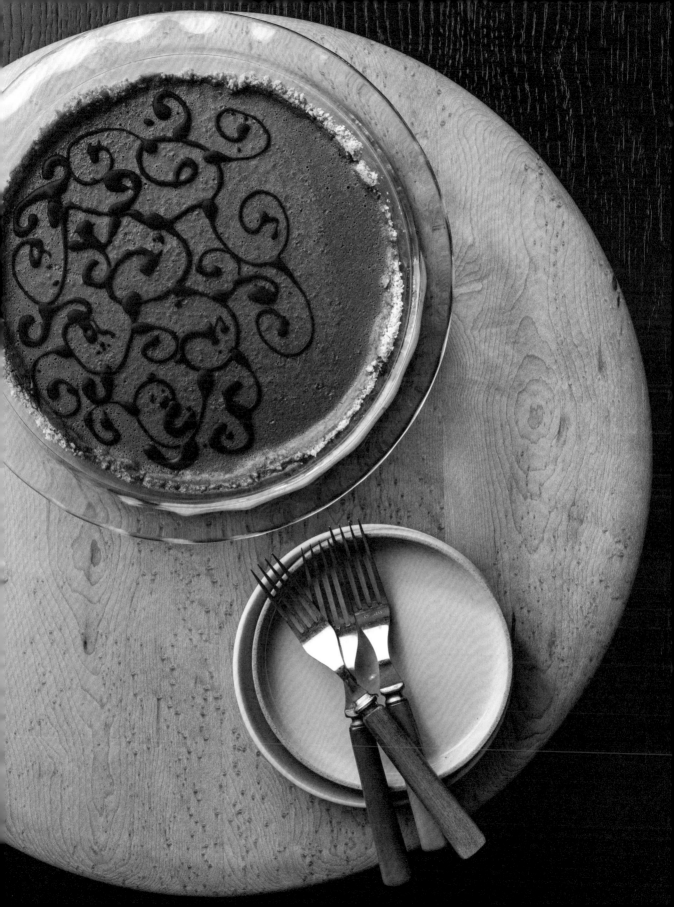

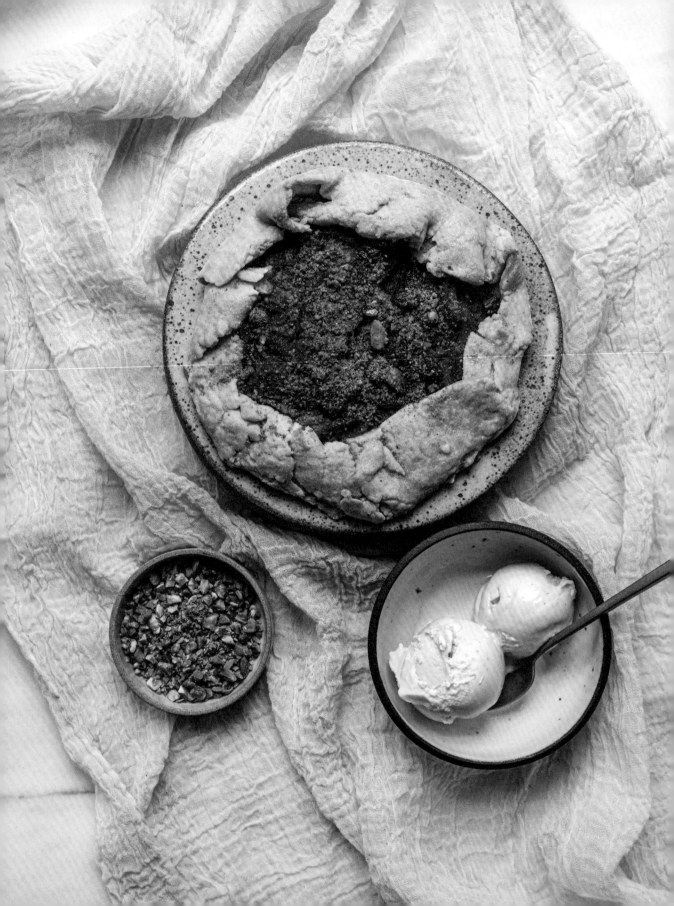

whatever you've got galette

This is a great way to use fresh fruits that appear to be on their last legs. And you could say it's as easy as pie. Once they've been boiled down they're revived into a delicious jam and held strong with chia seeds, a great way to get fiber, quality protein, and massive nutrients in a small serving.

———— MAKES ONE 9-INCH (23-CM) GALETTE (ABOUT 9 SERVINGS) ————

1 store-bought vegan piecrust

2 cups (400 g) any sort of fruit or berries (chopped strawberries, blueberries, apples, peaches, rhubarb are all excellent)

3½ tablespoons maple syrup

3 tablespoons coconut sugar, plus more for sprinkling

2 tablespoons chia seeds

1 teaspoon pure vanilla extract

135 milligrams CBD oil

Ice cream for serving (optional)

Preheat the oven to 350° F (180° C).

Roll out the dough for the piecrust according to instructions and place in a pie pan or on a baking sheet.

In a small saucepan over medium-low heat, combine the chopped fruit of your choice with the maple syrup, coconut sugar, chia seeds, and vanilla. Heat until fully dissolved, like chutney, and then allow to cool slightly. Spoon the filling in the center of the dough, leaving a 2-inch (5-cm) border. Fold the edges of the dough up and over the filling.

Sprinkle the assembled pie with coconut sugar and bake until the crust browns slightly and the filling bubbles, 12 to 17 minutes. Remove and promptly dose with the CBD oil (as the pie cools the oil will be absorbed). Allow the galette to cool before slicing and serve plain or with ice cream.

(V)

peanut butter pretzel pie

I'm not even going to attempt to pass this recipe off as particularly healthy, but it is vegan and leans toward conscious, healthy eating. It started as a birthday treat request for a friend but it turns out peanut butter and pretzels are universally enjoyed.

─── **MAKES ONE 9-INCH (23-CM) PIE (ABOUT 9 SERVINGS)** ───

FOR THE CRUST:

4 ounces (40 g) pretzels

¾ cup (30 g) Peanut Butter Puffins cereal

½ cup (100 g) cultured vegan butter (page 28)

FOR THE FILLING:

1 (13.5-ounce / 380-ml) can coconut milk

1 cup (180 g) chocolate chips

¾ cup (195 g) peanut butter

¼ cup (60 ml) maple syrup

½ cup (65 g) coconut sugar

2 teaspoons agar-agar flakes

135 milligrams CBD oil

Store-bought coconut cream, hot fudge (page 168), and pretzel crisps, for serving (optional)

Preheat the oven to 350° F (180° C).

Make the crust: In a food processor, blend the pretzels and cereal quickly (about 30 seconds), leaving some chunks. In a small saucepan over low heat, melt the butter, and then combine with the pretzels and cereal. Press mixture into a 9-inch (23-cm) pie pan and bake for 8 to 10 minutes, checking to make sure it doesn't burn. The crust will be slightly darker due to the pretzel coloring, but watch for a deepened brown to indicate it's ready to come out of the oven. Remove from the oven and allow to cool.

Make the filling: In a medium saucepan over low heat, combine the coconut milk with the chocolate chips, stirring. Once the chips have melted, add the peanut butter, maple syrup, coconut sugar, agar-agar flakes, and CBD oil; remove from the heat. Refrigerate the entire pan until the filling is no longer warm to the touch and has thickened slightly.

Spoon the filling into the piecrust and smooth over the top with a spatula. Cover the pie and refrigerate for 2 to 4 hours before slicing and serving.

For the optional garnishes, freeze the can of coconut cream for 2 hours, and then whip in a stand mixer for 1 to 2 minutes, and spoon onto the pie cold. Drizzle hot fudge and broken pretzel crisps.

(V)

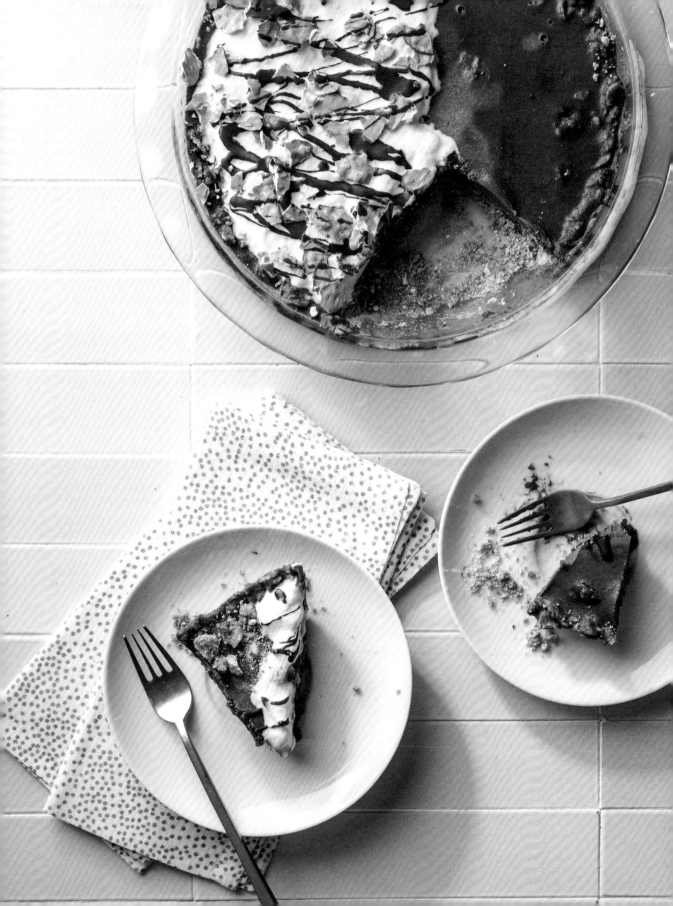

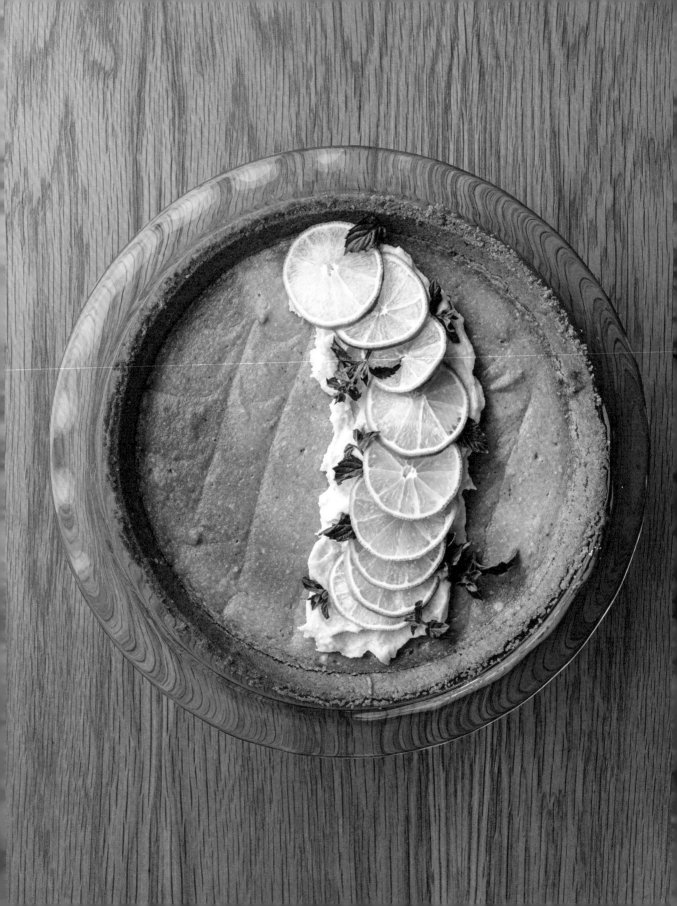

key lime pie

This is the best summer BBQ recipe. I say that because it's quick and easy if you need it to be. You can purchase ready-made yogurt if you don't have time to make your own, and you can use a store-bought graham cracker crust (check to make sure it's vegan if that matters). Psyllium also can lower blood sugar and is heart-healthy, working in this recipe as a bonding agent to hold the pie together.

—————— MAKES ONE 9-INCH (23-CM) PIE (ABOUT 9 SERVINGS) ——————

2 cups (300 g) raw cashews

1 cup (130 g) coconut sugar

½ cup (120 ml) coconut milk

2 tablespoons psyllium husk fiber

2 teaspoons lemon zest

2 teaspoons lime zest

¼ cup (60 ml) lime juice

1 teaspoon pure vanilla extract

½ teaspoon spirulina powder

135 milligrams CBD oil

1 (9-inch / 23-cm) gluten-free, store-bought graham cracker crust

Preheat the oven to 350° F (180° C).

In a high-speed blender, combine the cashews, coconut sugar, coconut milk, psyllium husk fiber, lemon and lime zest, lime juice, vanilla, spirulina powder, and the CBD oil with ½ cup water on high for 2 minutes; pour into the crust. Bake for 30 to 40 minutes, until the filling no longer jiggles but holds firm when touched. Allow to cool to room temp before transferring to fridge to chill for at leaset 2 hours before serving.

GF

puddings & ice creams

CHAPTER SEVEN

peanut butter chocolate pudding

Sometimes the simplest things are the best. This pudding can be made in seconds and it's always everyone's favorite. You can also freeze it for an ice cream, but I think it's best as a chilled pudding.

SERVES 2

½ cup (90 g) chocolate chips

1 (13.5-ounce / 380-ml) can coconut milk

½ cup (130 g) peanut butter

1 teaspoon pure vanilla extract

¼ teaspoon sea salt

½ tablespoon ashwagandha root powder

30 milligrams CBD oil

In a small saucepan over low heat, gently heat chocolate chips, stirring continuously until soft. Add the coconut milk, peanut butter, and vanilla and continue to stir until fully incorporated and smooth. Add the salt and remove from the heat, stirring in the ashwagandha until mixed. Refrigerate for at least 2 hours before spooning the pudding into bowls and dosing each with 15 milligrams CBD oil.

GF

V

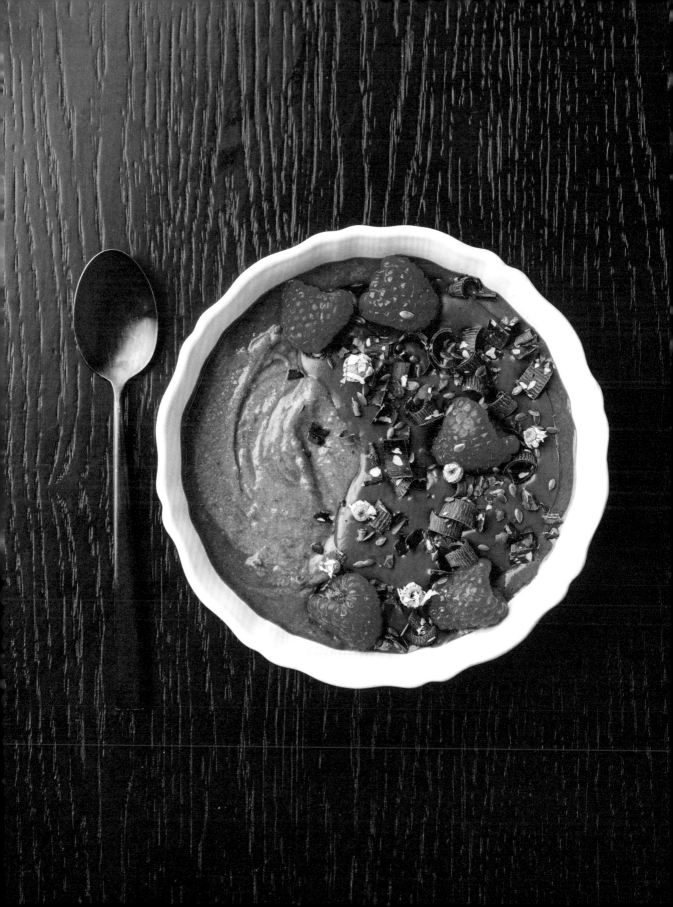

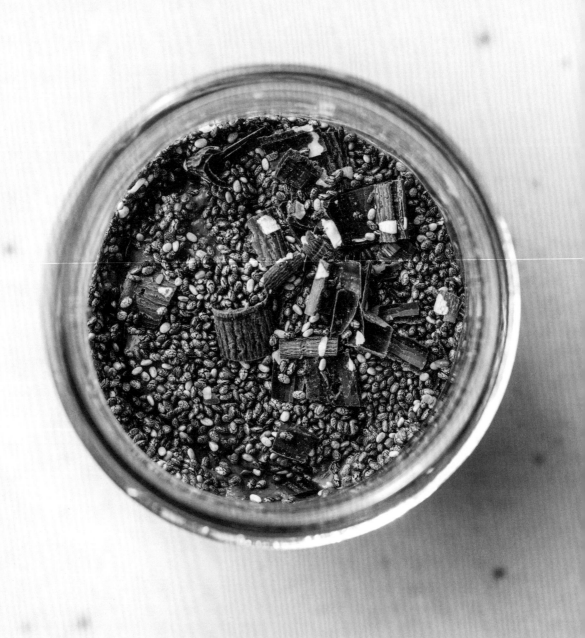

chocolate chia pudding

This is an early-morning favorite. Chia puddings are great because you make them the night before (or a few nights before) and they're waiting for you when you're still bleary-eyed and dazed. This one's extra great because it has maca root to give you a boost of energy and mental awareness, which I usually need first thing.

──────── SERVES 2 ────────

¾ cup (180 ml) cashew milk (page 20)

4 dates, pitted

2 tablespoons cocoa powder

2 tablespoons chia seeds

½ tablespoon maca root powder

¼ teaspoon pure vanilla extract

30 milligrams CBD oil

Granola (page 75), cacao nibs, or chocolate curls, for serving (optional)

In a high-speed blender, combine the cashew milk, dates, cocoa powder, chia seeds, maca powder, and vanilla, and blend on high for 2 to 3 minutes. Divide the mixture between 2 (8-ounce / 235-ml) mason jars, dosing each jar with 15 milligrams CBD oil, then refrigerate overnight or up to 5 days. I like to top these with granola and cacao nibs or chocolate curls.

GF

V

banana pudding

My family is Southern and one of my best friends is, too. The other day she asked me about a Southern-style banana pudding. Traditionally, it is filled with lady fingers, egg whites, and lots of cream, but this version is cashew cream–based with some lemon zest, maple syrup, and a crumbly almond meal crust layered with fresh banana, trifle-style. It's hardly a compromise—just delicious.

SERVES 9

FOR THE COOKIE CRUST:
½ cup (100 g) cultured vegan butter (page 28)
2 cups (170 g) almond flour
¼ cup (35 g) coconut sugar
2 tablespoons maple syrup
1 teaspoon pure vanilla extract
1 teaspoon almond extract

FOR THE BANANA PUDDING:
2 cups (300 g) raw cashews
12 ripe bananas
1 lemon, zested and juiced
3 tablespoons maple syrup
1 teaspoon pure vanilla extract
¼ teaspoon sea salt
135 milligrams CBD oil
2 bananas, thinly sliced for topping

Preheat the oven to 350° F (180° C). Line a baking sheet with parchment paper.

Make the cookie crust: In a saucepan over medium heat, brown the cultured vegan butter; remove from the heat. In a large mixing bowl, loosely combine the melted butter, almond flour, coconut sugar, maple syrup, vanilla, and almond extract.

Using clean hands, turn out the dough onto the parchment-lined baking sheet and flatten with your hands into a rustic, flat shape. (You'll break it apart later so don't fret about how it looks). Bake for 12 minutes, until it browns at the edges and holds firm and allow the crust to cool.

Make the pudding: In a high-speed blender, blend the cashews with the bananas, lemon juice and zest, maple syrup, vanilla, salt, and CBD oil. Blend on high for 2 minutes, then scrape down the sides and blend for 30 seconds more.

Assemble the pudding: Using your hands, crumble up the cooled cookie and start layering the pudding into 9 small glass cups or bowls. Start with a layer of the cookie crust. Top with some banana slices, followed by pudding. Smooth with a spoon before adding another layer of cookie crust followed by more banana (the banana is more to provide texture than for looks, it can be scant or randomly placed) and pudding and then finish off each individual parfait with more cookie crust on top. Enjoy immediately.

GF
V

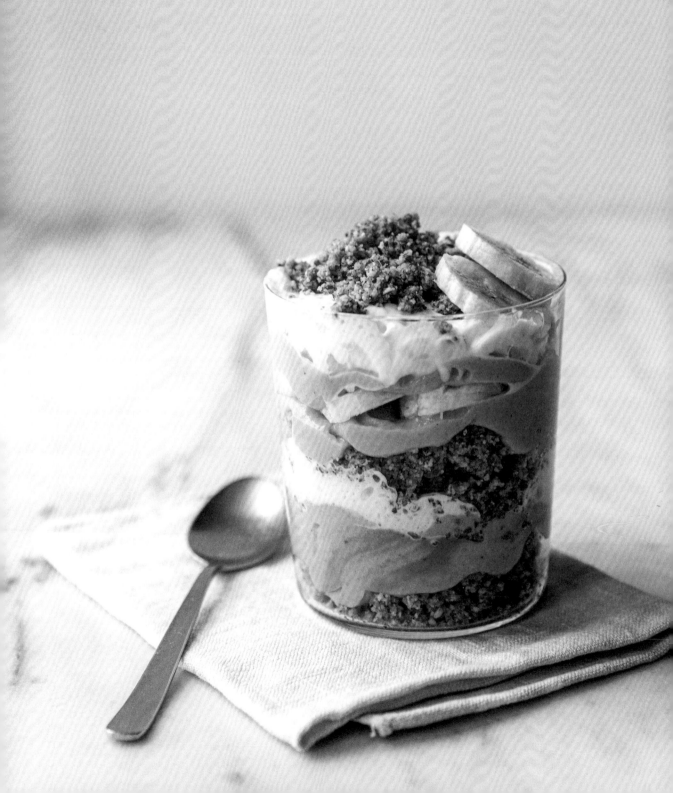

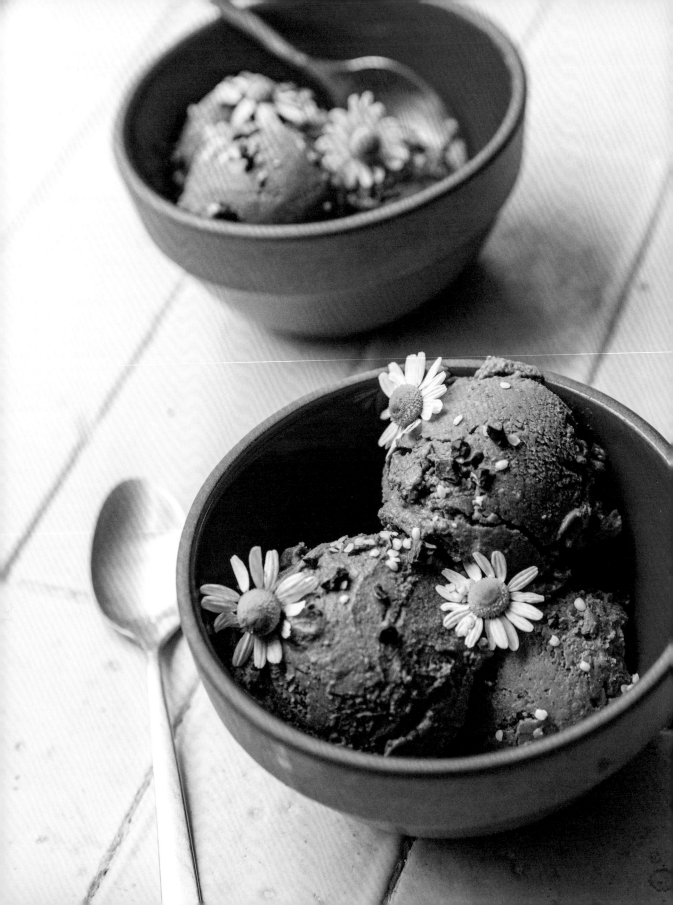

chocolate almond butter ice cream

Nobody ever tells you how easy ice cream is to make. Really, even without an ice cream maker (although those are indisputably more fun), ice cream is a snap. All you need is a freezer and some patience, plus you can avoid all the weird additives most ice creams come with when you buy them from the store.

—————————————— SERVES 4 ——————————————

4 ounces (95 g) dark vegan chocolate, coarsely chopped

1 (13.5-ounce / 380-ml) can coconut milk

2 tablespoons almond butter

2 tablespoons coconut butter (page 25)

¼ cup (60 ml) maple syrup

1 teaspoon *Mucuna pruriens* powder

1 teaspoon pure vanilla extract

140 milligrams CBD oil

In a small saucepan over medium-low heat, gently heat the chocolate and coconut milk slowly to incorporate (do not bring to a boil). Add the almond butter, coconut butter, and maple syrup, and remove from the heat. Allow to cool for 5 to 10 minutes before adding the Mucuna pruriens, vanilla, and CBD oil.

Transfer the entire mixture to a freezer-safe, lidded dish and freeze for 4 to 6 hours, stirring every hour. Alternatively, use an ice cream maker and allow to process for 30 minutes before transferring to a freezer-safe, lidded dish; allow to set for 4 to 6 hours before serving.

Note: Dairy-free ice cream can be difficult to scoop. If you really want beautiful rounds of ice cream, allow to soften slightly prior to serving, 10 minutes or so.

(GF)

(V)

sauces, icings
& toppings

hot fudge

This hot fudge dresses up any recipe and makes it a little more special. It's also a great way to add CBD to anything that might not have included it to start.

──────── **MAKES ABOUT 1 CUP (240 ML)** ────────

½ cup (90 g) chocolate chips

2 tablespoons nut butter

60 milligrams CBD oil

In a small saucepan over low to medium heat, melt both the chocolate and nut butter, stirring gently until combined. Do not overheat or bring to a boil; remove from the heat once combined, adding CBD oil once slightly cooled.

Pictured right, in the small white pitcher.

GF
V

caramel sauce

This caramel sauce works as a frosting, dipping sauce, or ice cream topper. I like it warm, but it's great at any temperature.

──────── **MAKES ABOUT 1 CUP (240 ML)** ────────

2 tablespoons cultured vegan butter (page 28), at room temperature

5 dates, pitted

½ cup (120 ml) coconut cream (solids only, not the watery layer)

2 tablespoons nut butter

1 teaspoon sea salt

120 milligrams CBD oil

In a high-speed blender, combine the vegan butter, dates, coconut cream, nut butter, salt and the CBD oil. Blend on high for 2 to 3 minutes, adding warm water by tablespoonfuls to reach desired thickness. (For a glaze I will add a few tablespoons of water; for a more sticky toffee caramel sauce I won't add any at all.)

Pictured right, in the bright blue bowl.

GF
V

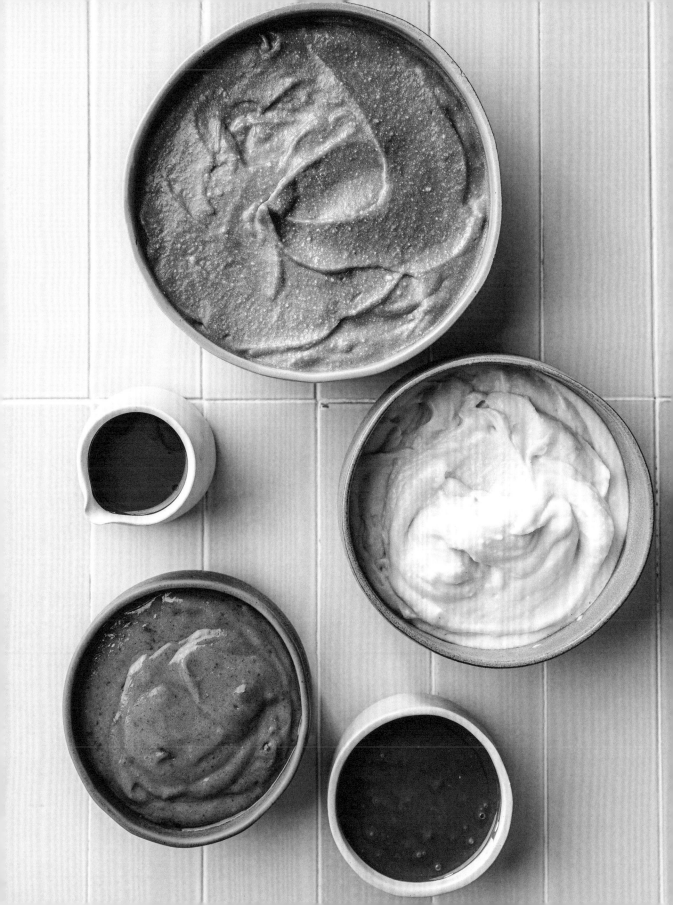

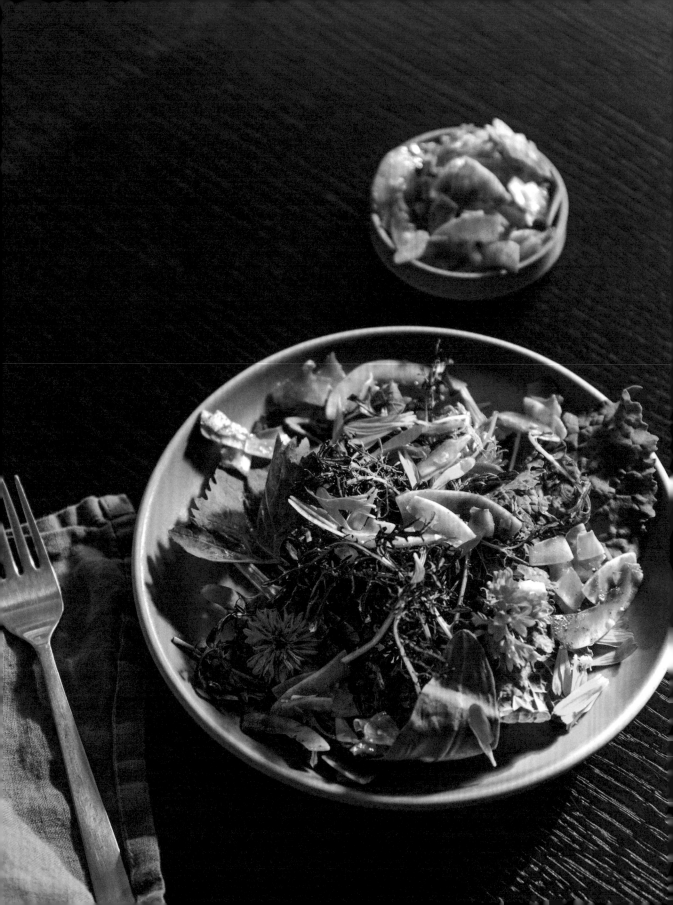

coconut bacon

We use this for both sweets and savories: it's a nice crunch on salad but makes for the perfect salty-sweet flavor on cupcakes and ice cream, too. It's wonderful on cakes—you can pile it high as an addition to any frosting.

―――――――――― **MAKES ABOUT 2 CUPS (200 G)** ――――――――――

2 cups (200 g) dried coconut (both sweetened and unsweetened work but I use unsweetened and a large flake; shredded sweetened coconut is decadent and more dessert-like)

1 tablespoon avocado oil

2 tablespoons liquid aminos (soy sauce and tamari also work)

1 tablespoon maple syrup

¼ teaspoon liquid smoke

½ teaspoon sea salt

240 milligrams CBD oil

Preheat the oven to 350° F (180° C). Line a baking sheet with parchment paper.

In a large bowl, stir together the coconut, avocado oil, liquid aminos, maple syrup, liquid smoke, and salt until the coconut is completely coated. Spread the coconut evenly across the baking sheet.

Bake for 8 minutes, then check on it and give it a stir if some bits are darkening faster than others. Continue to bake until it's browned a bit, about 6 to 10 minutes more. Let the "bacon" cool for several minutes so it has a chance to crisp up a bit.

(GF)

(V)

maple coconut butter

I use this on pancakes and toast and it's always a hit when we go camping—a quick way to deliver CBD to almost anything and easy to carry premade.

——— **MAKES ABOUT ¾ CUP (180 ML)** ———

½ cup (100 g) cultured vegan butter (page 28), melted

¼ teaspoon pure vanilla extract

2 tablespoons maple syrup

120 milligrams CBD oil

In a small dish lined with parchment paper, combine all the ingredients (butter, vanilla, maple syrup, CBD oil). Each serving, at this 12-milligram dose, is 2 tablespoons. Distribute accordingly.

Refrigerate for at least 6 hours, until resolidified, and use as you would butter.

Pictured right, in the bright blue bowl.

GF

V

peanut butter chocolate sauce

I use this as a ganache when hardened and as a sauce when warm. It's good drizzled on anything—sugar cookies, ice cream, you name it. And it coats granola bars, energy bites, and even pretzels perfectly.

——— **MAKES 1¼ CUPS (300 ML)** ———

1 cup (180 g) chocolate chips

¼ cup (65 g) peanut butter

120 milligrams CBD oil

In a small saucepan over low heat, heat the chocolate chips and peanut butter, stirring continuously. Add the CBD oil and remove from the heat. Each serving, at this 12 milligram dose, is 2 tablespoons. Distribute accordingly. The mixture will harden if cooled (which is great on pretzels or when used as a ganache).

Pictured right, in the small white bowl.

GF

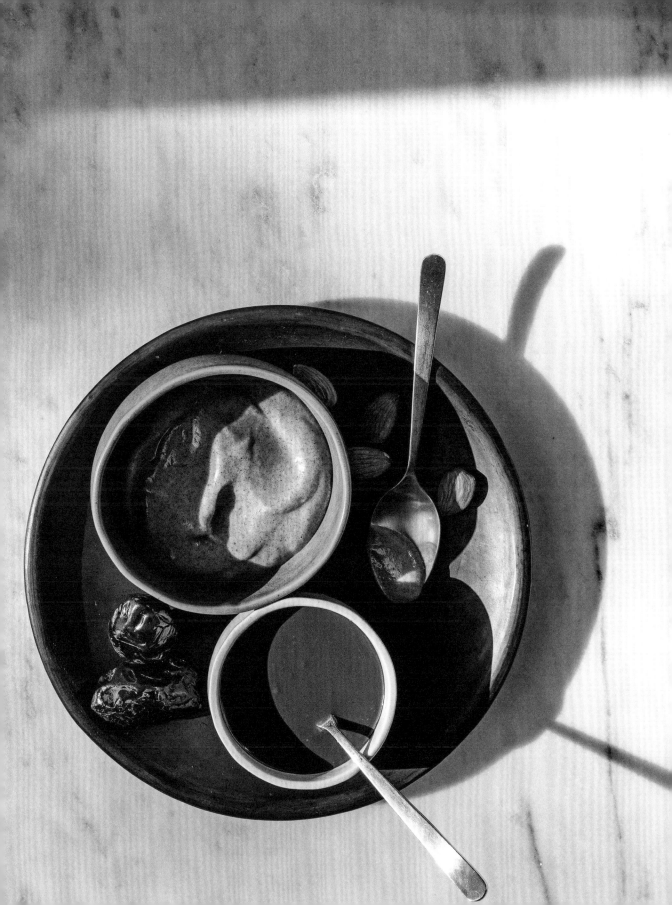

vanilla frosting

This is the most versatile frosting ever: You can add chocolate, or peanut butter, to mix up the flavors, or use a tiny bit of turmeric, spirulina, or freeze-dried strawberries for color. I use this on the carrot cake and sprinkle it with coconut. It also works on the Almond, Rosemary, and Olive Oil Cake (page 136) with lemon zest. It does contain confectioner's sugar, since any other sugar is too heavy and will make it gritty or chunky. Maple syrup will make it runny, more like a glaze, but if refined sugars aren't your thing give it a shot.

MAKES 1 CUP (240 ML)

1 cup (90 g) confectioner's sugar

1 cup (200 g) cultured vegan butter (page 28), at room temperature

½ teaspoon pure vanilla extract

120 milligrams CBD oil

Sift the confectioner's sugar and set aside.

In the bowl of a stand mixer, add room temperature cultured vegan butter and vanilla extract, beating on low for about 30 seconds. Scrape down the sides of the bowl with a rubber spatula and then add the sifted confectioner's sugar, a few tablespoons at a time, stopping to run the mixer at short intervals (about 30 seconds at a time), and scraping the sides down, too, until fully incorporated. Add in the CBD oil and mix by hand for another minute or two, fully scraping down the sides one more time before you use the frosting.

Picture page 169.

GF

V

chocolate frosting

I love this chocolate frosting because it firms up in the fridge and makes for the most stable cakes EVER. It's also amazingly simple and yummy.

———————— MAKES 1 CUP (240 ML) ————————

1 cup (180 g) chocolate chips

1 tablespoon coconut oil

1 cup (200 g) cultured vegan butter (page 28), at room temperature

120 milligrams CBD oil

In a small saucepan over low heat, melt the chocolate chips and coconut oil, stirring continuously. Remove from the heat and continue to stir, allowing the mixture to cool to room temperature. Once cool, transfer the chocolate mixture to the bowl of a stand mixer along with the softened butter and the CBD oil; mix to incorporate. The frosting will get thinner the warmer it gets so don't be afraid to give it a rest in the fridge. This is also great for icing a cake, because the frosting firms up quickly and works to hold the cake together nicely.

Picture page 169.

(GF)

(V)

savories

salsa verde

My mother-in-law is the best cook. She grew up in Mexico and all her recipes are delicious and fresh. As a bonus, she's always up to try anything I'm into, even if it's breaking from tradition—or not the way she'd do it if I weren't there. She was happy to omit the chicken stock for me and add just a pinch of salt instead.

—————————————— SERVES 4 ——————————————

5 tomatillos

1 cup (240 ml) vegetable broth

2 serrano peppers, stems trimmed and seeds removed (unless you want more spice)

1 bunch of cilantro

1 lime, zested and juiced

½ teaspoon sea salt

60 milligrams CBD oil

In a food processor, combine all the ingredients (tomatillos, vegetable broth, serrano peppers, cilantro, lime zest and juice, salt, and CBD oil) and blitz for 1 minute, leaving some of the texture. If you'd like a creamier version, you can also add ½ cup (120 ml) of cashew cream (page 27). This recipe contains 15 milligrams CBD oil per (2 tablespoon) serving.

GF

V

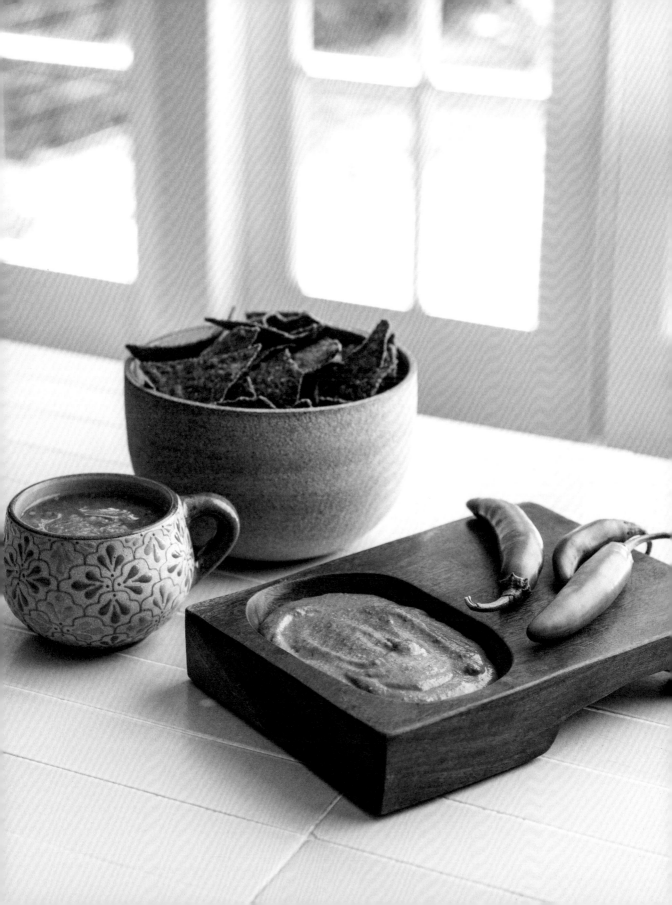

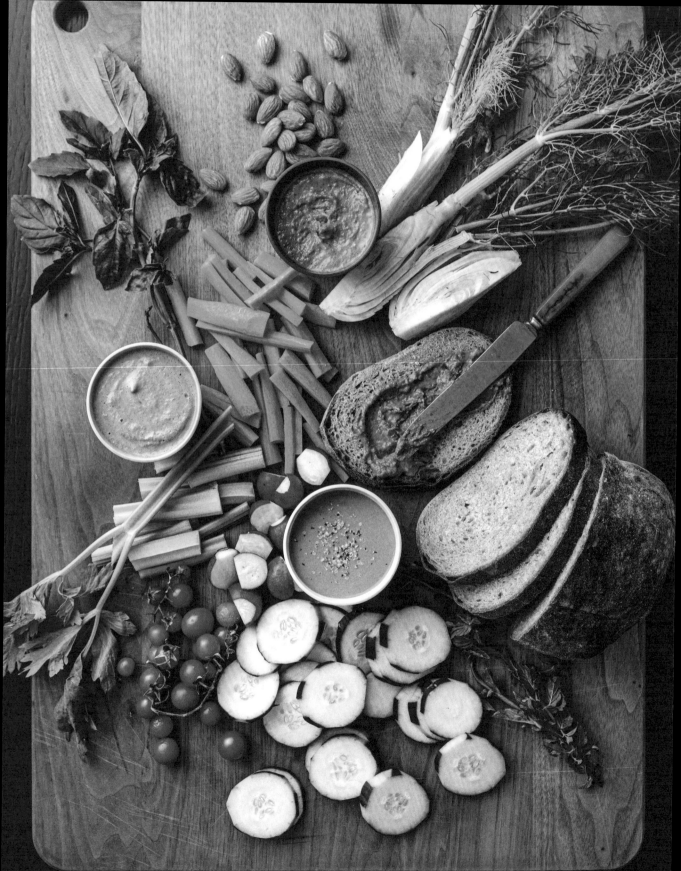

basil and hemp seed pesto

When I first began making food for others, there was an influx of people who weren't into sweets: They couldn't eat them, didn't want them, and didn't like them. Savory sauces and dressings are a great way to eat CBD with a fat. The hemp seed pesto is my favorite complement to hemp-based CBD.

SERVES 8

3 cups (90 g) fresh basil leaves

¼ cup (40 g) hemp seeds

2 lemons, juiced

¼ cup (60 ml) extra virgin olive oil

2 cloves garlic

2 tablespoons nutritional yeast

1 teaspoon sea salt

120 milligrams CBD oil

In a high-speed blender, combine all the ingredients (basil, hemp seeds, lemon juice, olive oil, garlic, nutritional yeast, and sea salt) except the CBD oil and blend on high for 2 to 3 minutes. Once everything is mixed and you have a pesto, gently stir the CBD oil into the pesto. Serve over pasta, salads, or tomatoes and cheese for a caprese-style salad. This recipe contains 15 milligrams CBD oil per (1 tablespoon) serving.

GF

V

caesar dressing

I really love using the Best Buds for Life CBD oil in savory recipes. This CBD oil has a unique flavor and smooth texture that lends itself to a creamy dressing. I use this on massaged kale and usually add avocado and toasted nuts on top.

———————————————— SERVES 4 ————————————————

½ cup (120 ml) cashew cream (page 27)

2 lemons, zested and juiced

2 cloves garlic

1 tablespoon dijon mustard

2 tablespoons olive oil

3 tablespoons nutritional yeast

½ teaspoon soy sauce or tamari sauce

¼ teaspoon sea salt

½ teaspoon black pepper

60 milligrams CBD oil

In a high-speed blender, mix the cashew, lemon zest and juice, garlic, mustard, olive oil, nutritional yeast, soy or tamari sauce, salt, pepper, and CBD oil and blend for 2 to 3 minutes. This recipe contains 15 milligrams CBD oil per (2 tablespoon) serving.

GF

V

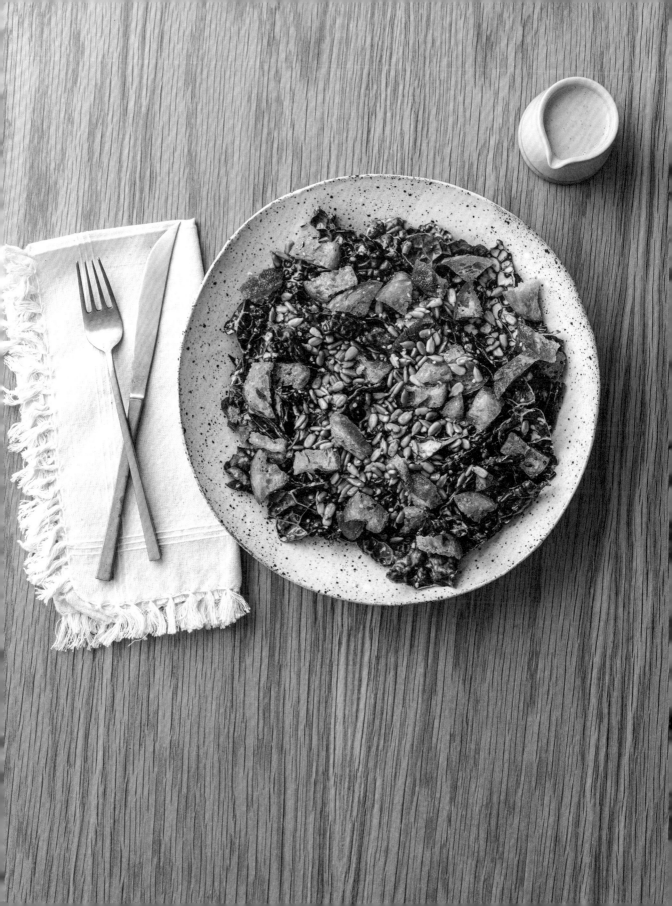

green goddess dressing

I make this at home all summer long while the garden is in full bloom. I list dill, parsley, and thyme, below, but really almost anything works, including holy basil, which it seems like everyone is into now. Use to dress a salad or dip veggies.

———— SERVES 4 ————

1 cup (150 g) raw cashews

2 lemons, zested and juiced

3 tablespoons chopped dill

1 tablespoon chopped parsley

½ tablespoon chopped thyme

2 tablespoons olive oil

2 tablespoons nutritional yeast

2 cloves garlic

60 milligrams CBD oil

In a high-speed blender, combine the cashews, lemon zest and juice, dill, parsley, thyme, olive oil, nutritional yeast, garlic, and CBD oil and blitz for 2 minutes until fully combined, adding 2 to 3 tablespoons of water as needed. This recipe contains 15 milligrams CBD oil per (2 tablespoon) serving.

GF

V

red pepper lazy girl romesco

I can't just call it romesco because real romesco has so much more going on.
This version, however, is delicious and simple, two things that I'm very into.
Great with crusty bread or as a dip.

SERVES 8

2 red peppers, cored and seeded

½ cup (75 g) raw almonds

2 cloves garlic

¼ cup (60 ml) avocado oil, for dousing

½ cup (120 ml) olive oil

2 tablespoons balsamic vinegar

120 milligrams CBD oil

Preheat the oven to 400° F (200° C). Line a baking sheet with parchment paper.

Combine the peppers, almonds, and garlic on the lined baking sheet and douse with a heat-safe oil (avocado oil has a high burn point and is generally my pick). Roast until everything has browned a bit, 12 to 15 minutes. In a food processor, combine all the roasted ingredients with the olive oil and balsamic vinegar and blend together for 1 minute. Scrape down the sides of the food processor and put into a bowl, adding the CBD oil and stirring carefully to distribute throughout.

GF

V

queso dip

I got an order for spinach artichoke dip a few months ago, and having never really eaten it I wasn't sure what to do. After a little experimentation I wound up with this. It's best served warm, and more queso-ish than spinach artichoke (mostly because, at the moment of inception I had harissa paste rather than artichokes on hand). I declare it a victory and its own thing.

SERVES 4

½ cup (75 g) raw cashews

3 tablespoons nutritional yeast

1 tablespoon onion powder

2 tablespoons harissa (chile pepper paste)

½ cup (15 g) fresh spinach

2 cloves garlic

¼ cup (60 ml) vegetable broth

60 milligrams CBD oil

In a high-speed blender, combine all the ingredients (cashews, nutritional yeast, onion powder, harissa, spinach, garlic, and vegetable broth) except the CBD oil and blend on high for 2 to 3 minutes. Scrape down the sides of the blender and put into a bowl and add the CBD oil, stirring to blend.

green gazpacho soup

I like this in summer when it's too hot to turn on a stove. It's crisp, seasonal, and so refreshing. We manage to grow nearly all the main ingredients in our home garden and you should try, too—they're nearly impossible to kill when the season's right, even when ignored regularly by the most absentminded gardener.

──── **SERVES 2** ────

1 avocado

½ cup (100 g) fresh corn kernels

½ cup (100 g) fresh tomatoes, chopped

2 tablespoons balsamic vinegar

1 small-to-medium cucumber, peeled

2 tablespoons fresh cilantro

1 teaspoon sea salt

1 teaspoon black pepper

½ cup (120 ml) vegetable broth

30 milligrams CBD oil

Cucumber and tomatoes, minced, for serving (optional)

In a high-speed blender, combine avocado, corn, tomatoes, balsamic vinegar, cucumber, cilantro, salt and pepper and blend on high for 2 minutes. Add the broth and mix for another 1 minute before dividing between bowls; garnish with cucumbers and tomatoes, if using, plus a swirl of 15 milligrams of CBD oil for each.

GF

V

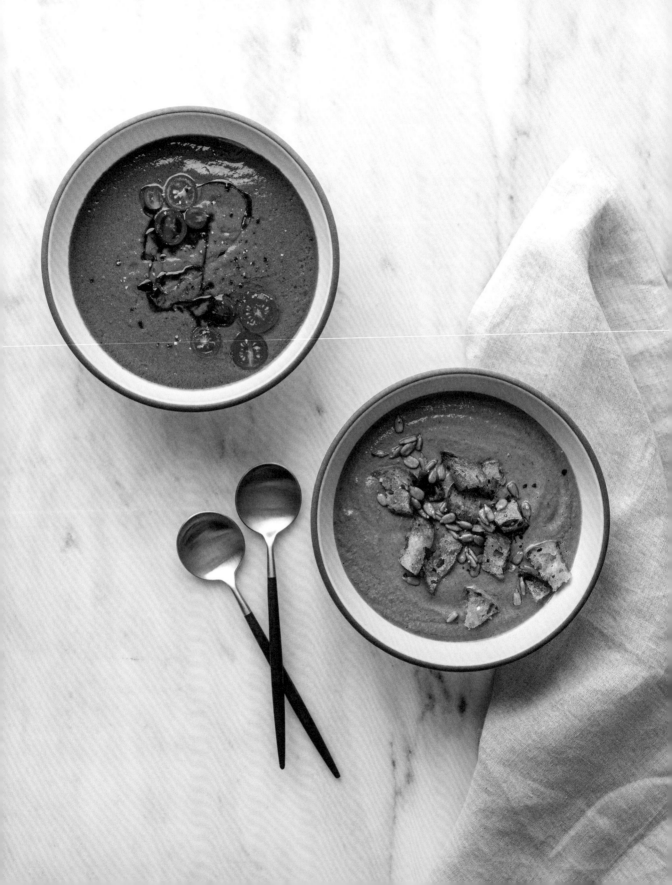

winter greens soup

In the winter, even in California, our garden situation is less diverse. Kale and Brussels sprouts are a sure thing, so this recipe was born. It's an especially great way to use leftover roasted greens from the night before. If you don't have leftovers you can just toss chopped veggies in a pan with a bit of salt and heat-safe oil for 10 to 15 minutes until lightly browned (or, as is often the case in my house, quite brown. I like them better this way).

I garnish the soup with toasted seeds and croutons—that is, the baguette I forgot to eat quickly enough or that my children left on their plates the day before, cubed and pan-fried in avocado oil with salt and pepper until brown and crisp. Boring old bread reborn as something new: a dinnertime phoenix miracle.

———————— SERVES 2 ————————

FOR THE SOUP:

1 cup plus 1 tablespoon (100 g) roasted Brussels sprouts, halved

1 cup plus 1 tablespoon (75 g) chopped, roasted kale

1 cup (150 g) raw cashews

1 cup (240 ml) vegetable broth

1 tablespoon balsamic vinegar

1 tablespoon nutritional yeast (plus 1 tablespoon for garnish)

FOR SERVING:

½ cup (30 g) cubed day-old baguette, for garnish

Olive oil

Sea salt

Freshly ground black pepper

30 milligrams CBD oil

½ cup (65 g) sunflower seeds, for garnish

Make the soup: In a high-speed blender, combine the Brussels sprouts, kale, cashews, vegetable broth, balsamic vinegar, and nutritional yeast and blend on high for 2 to 3 minutes, reserving an extra tablespoon each of kale and sprouts if you like a chunkier soup. Pour the blended soup into a heavy-bottomed pan (or cast-iron skillet for extra iron!) and warm on the stovetop until it reaches your desired temperature.

Prepare the toppings: While the soup heats up you can toast the sunflower seeds and fry the croutons (I do this in the same pan, because why wash multiples when you don't have to?) Add the cubed bread with some olive oil and salt and pepper first, stirring continuously until golden, then add the sunflower seeds for another minute.

Drizzle each bowl of soup with a swirl of 15 milligrams CBD oil and sprinkle with a handful of the toasted sunflower seeds and croutons.

(GF)

(V)

index